Section 1: Vata

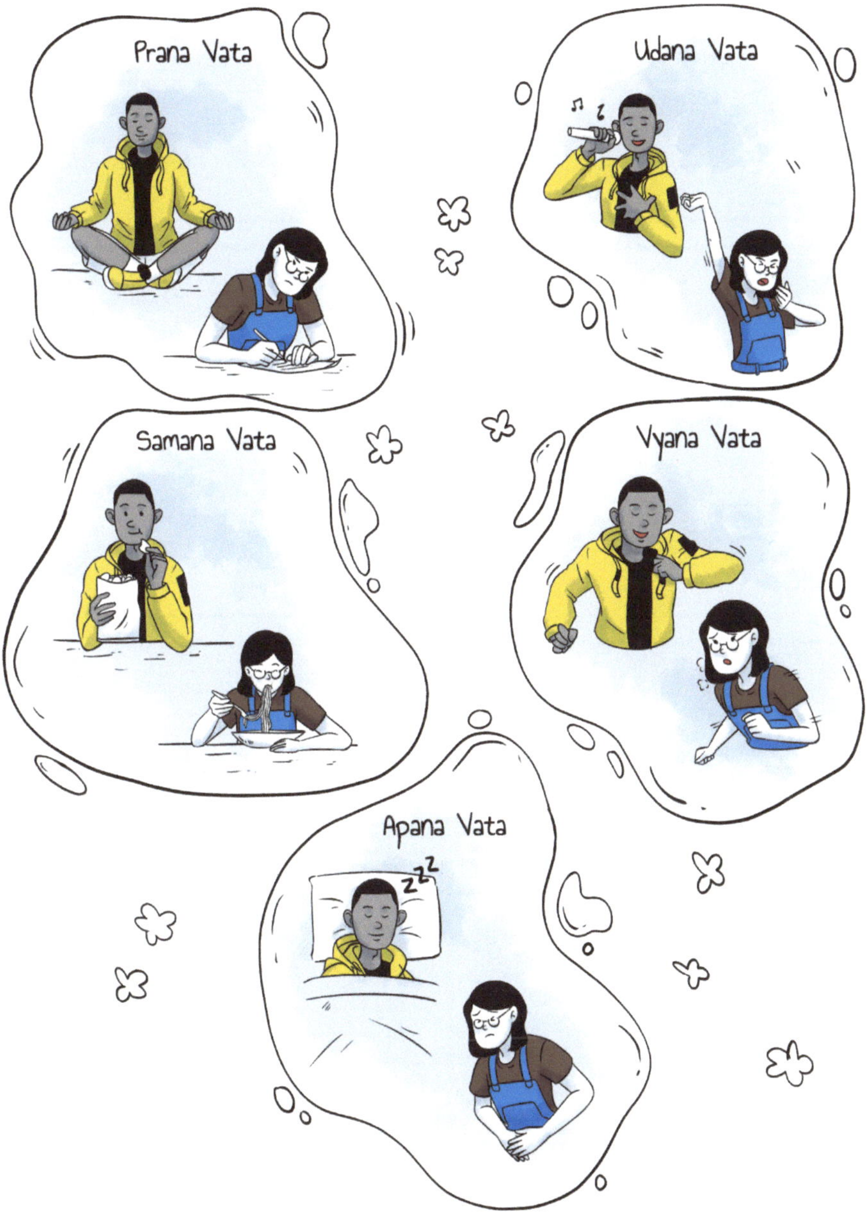

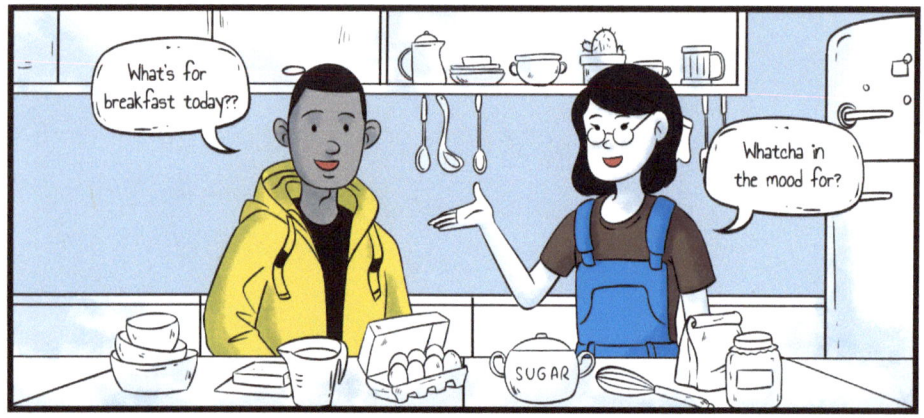
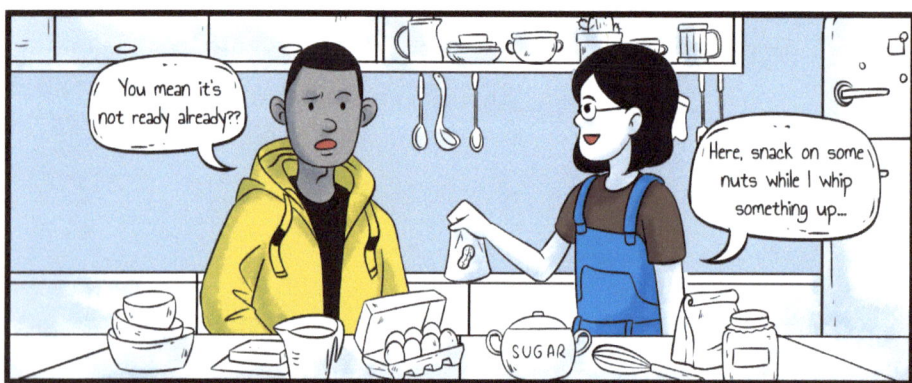
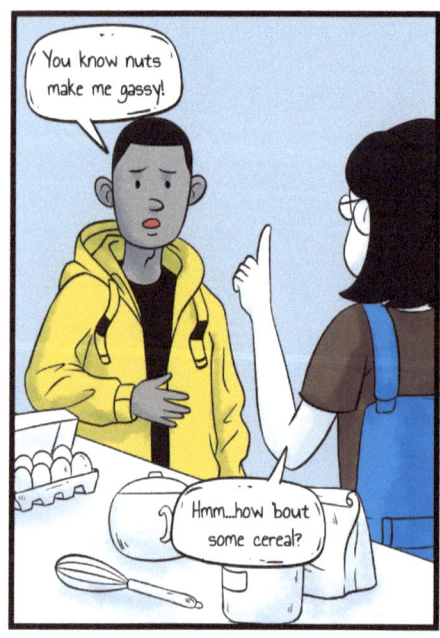
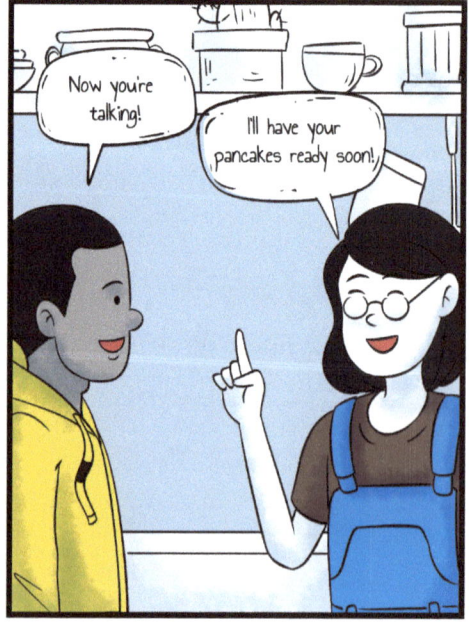

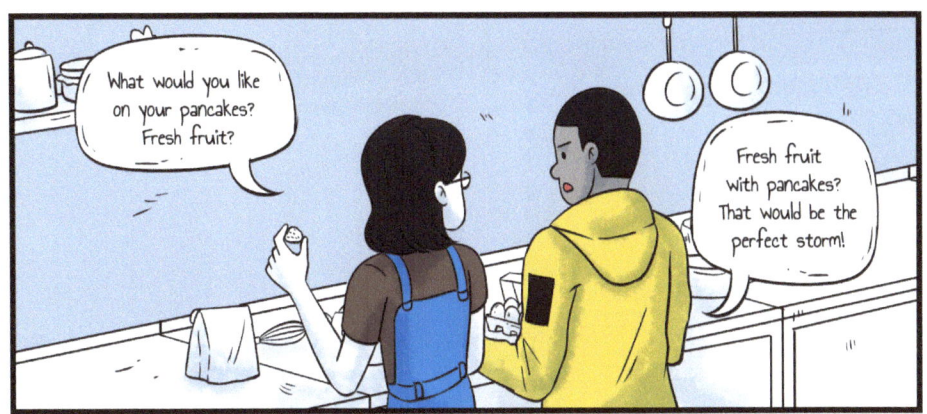

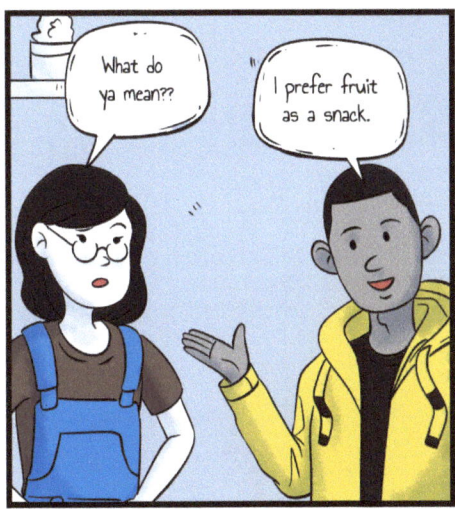

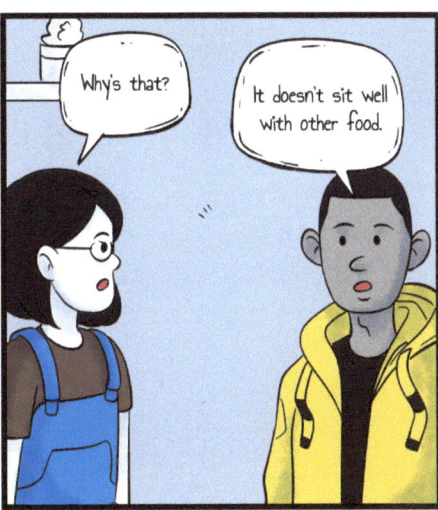

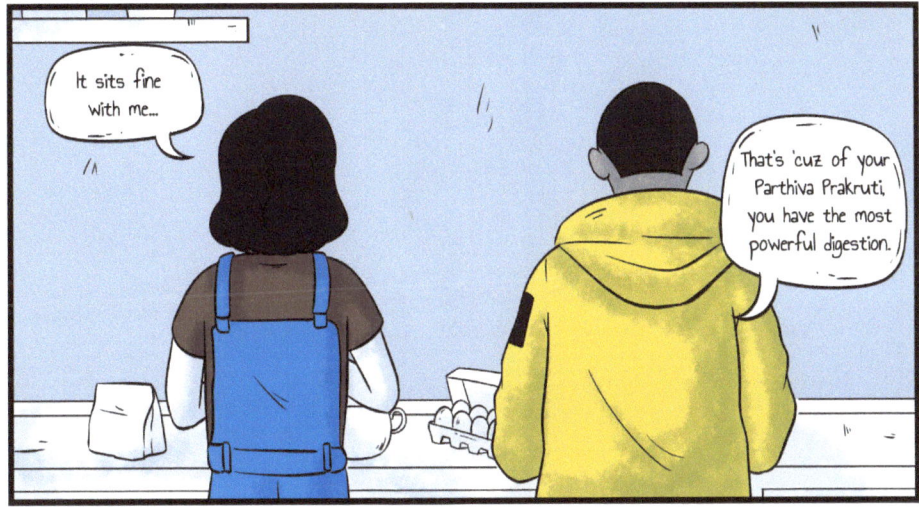

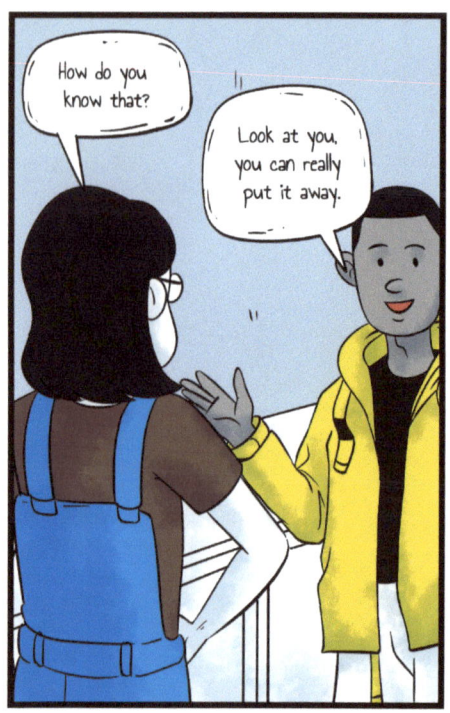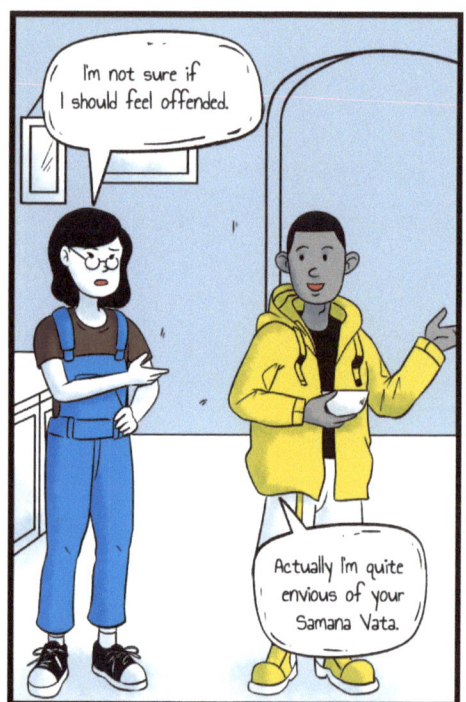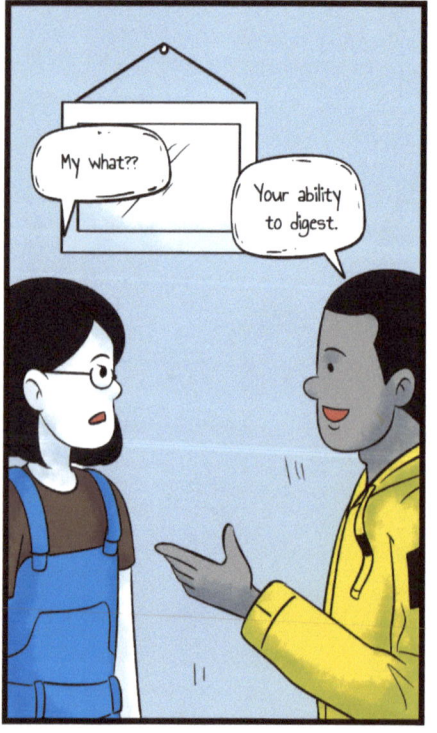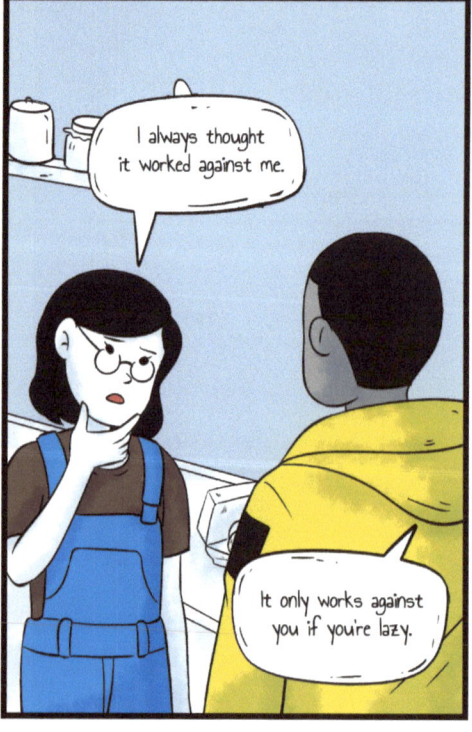

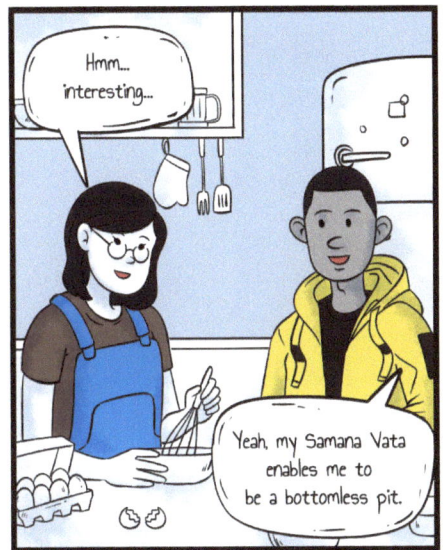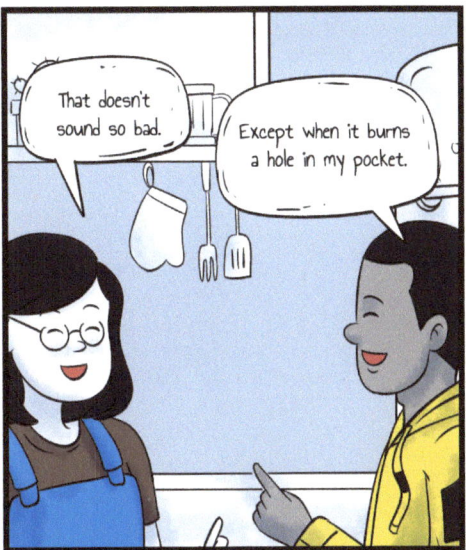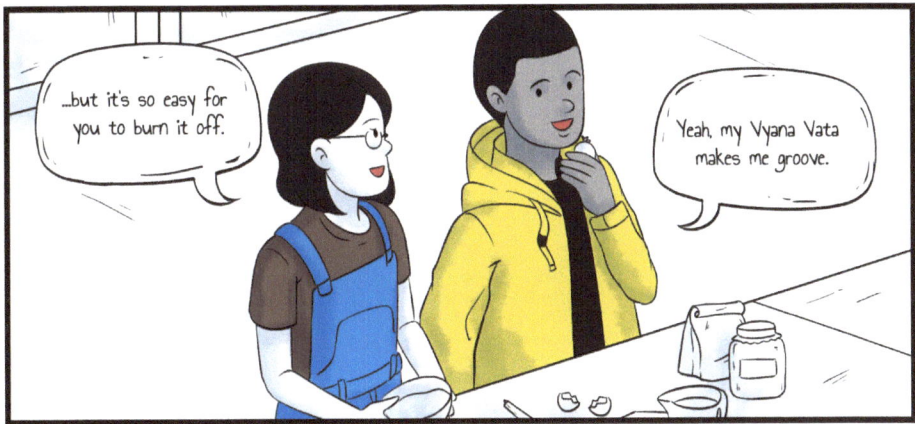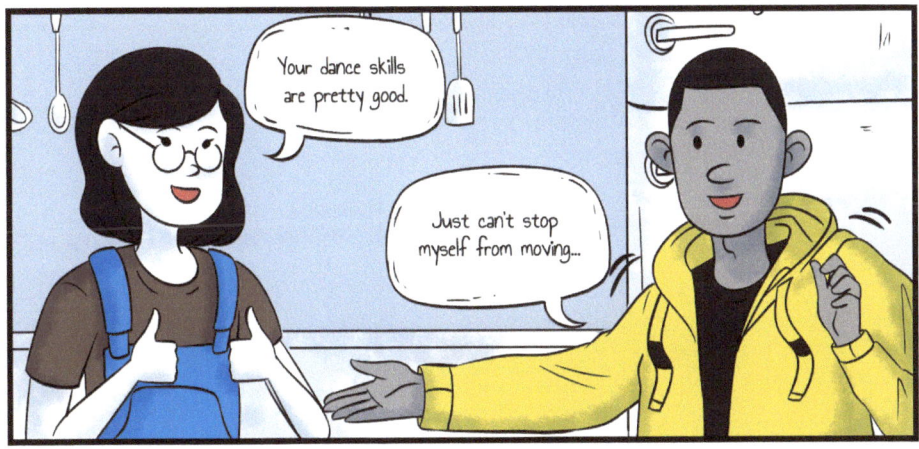

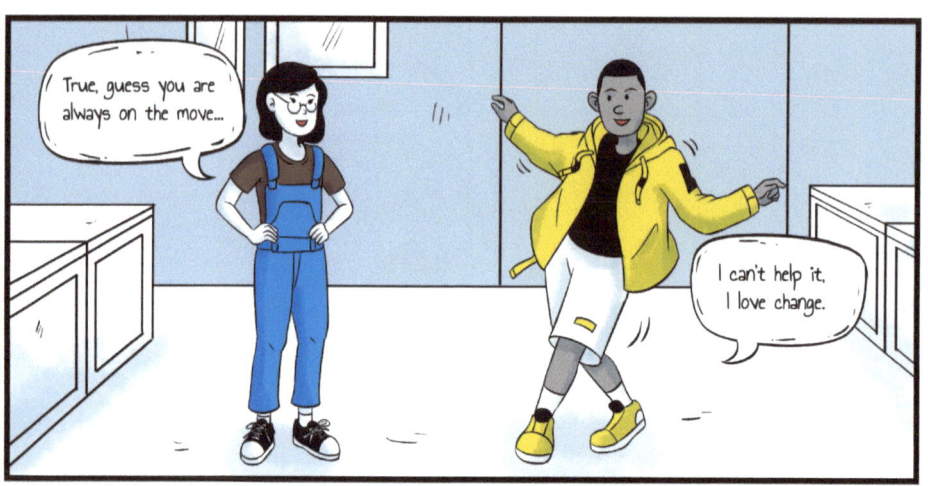
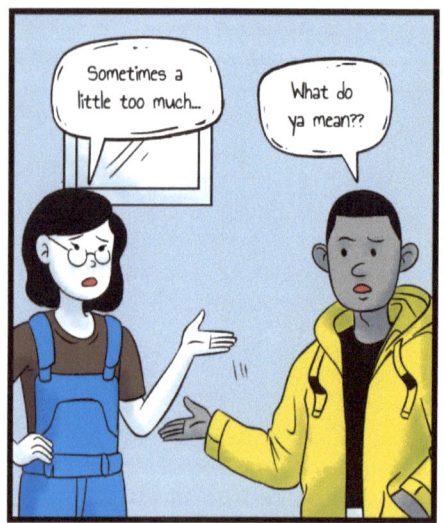
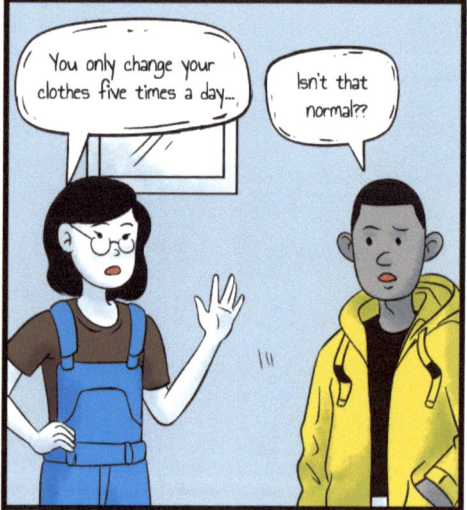
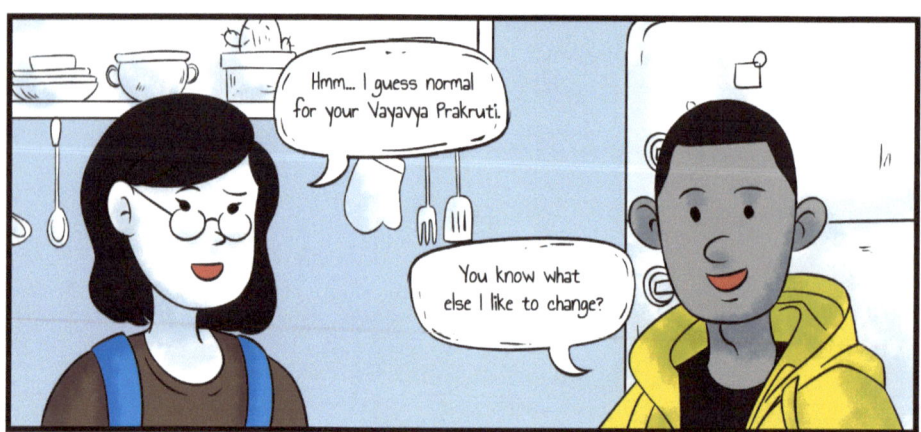

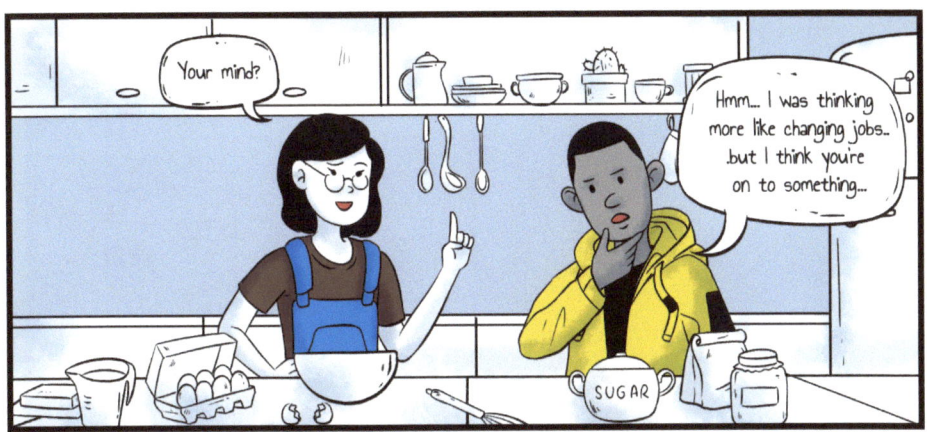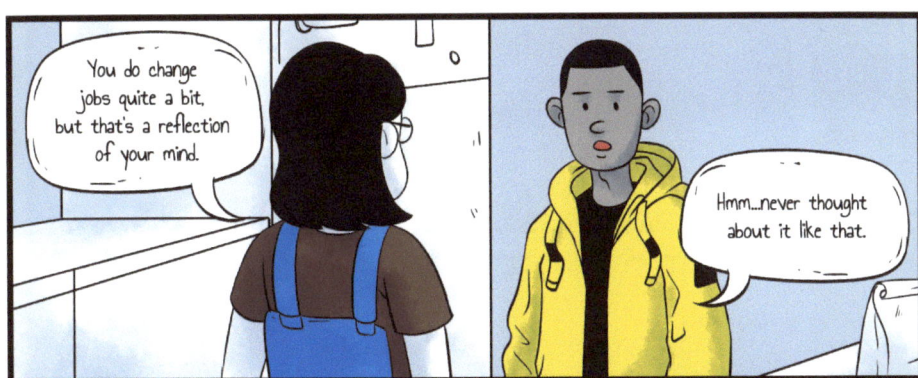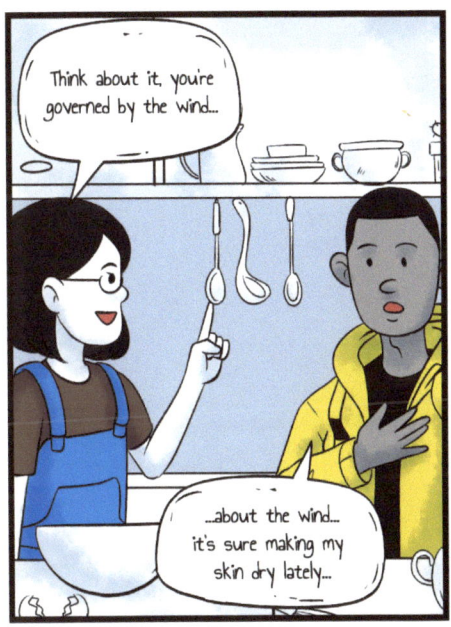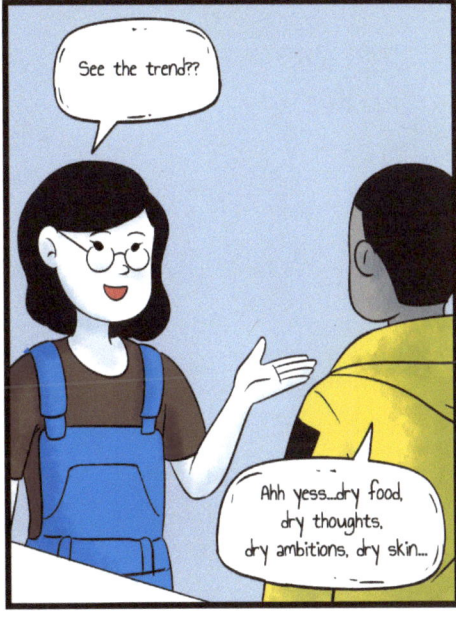

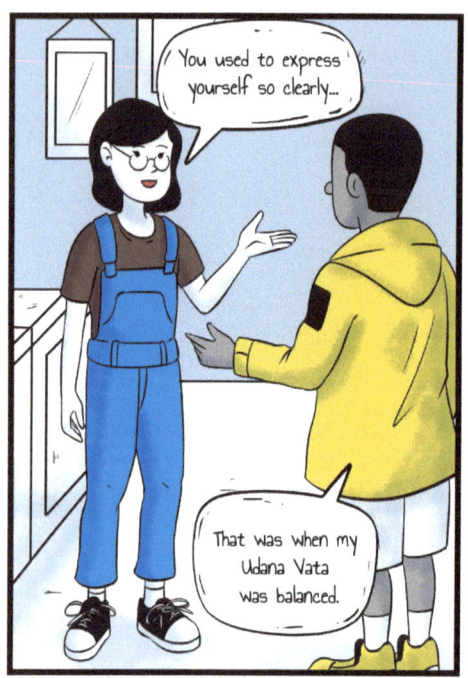
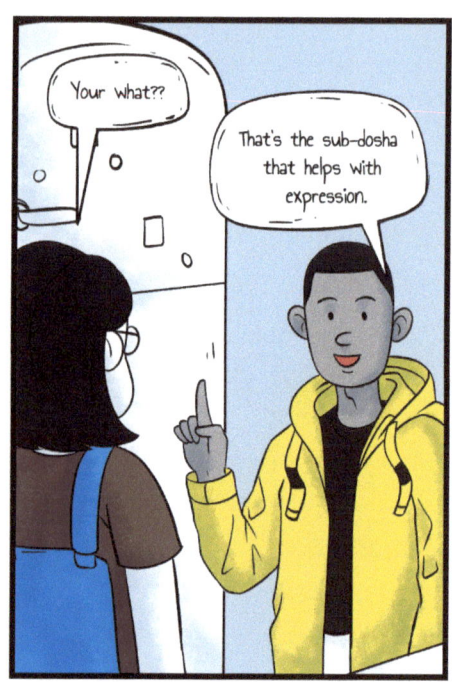
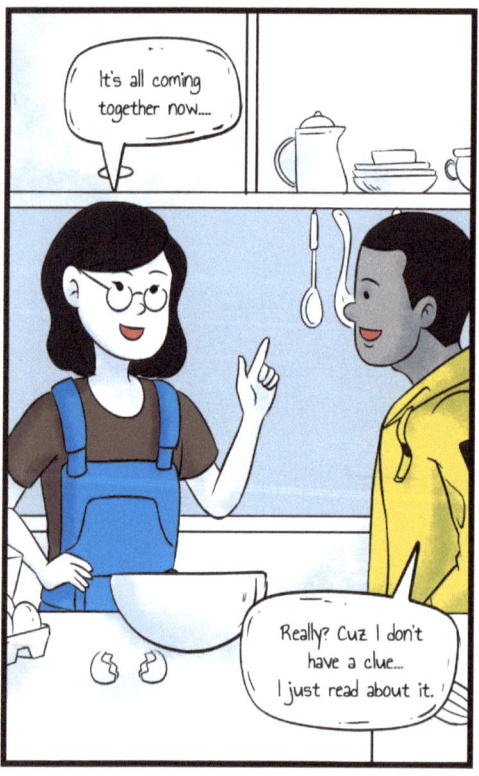
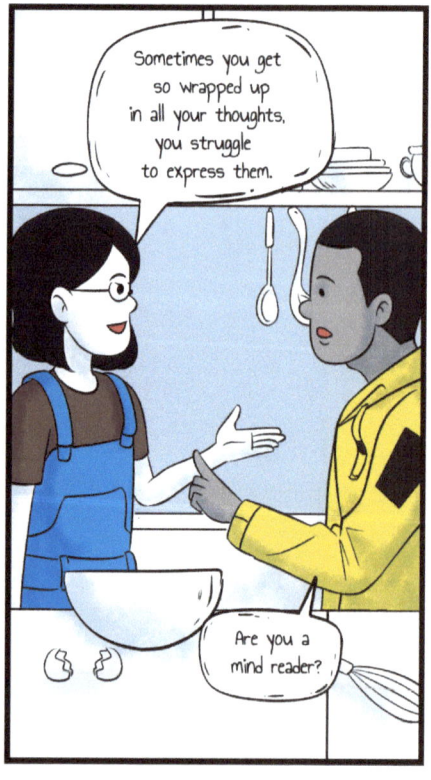

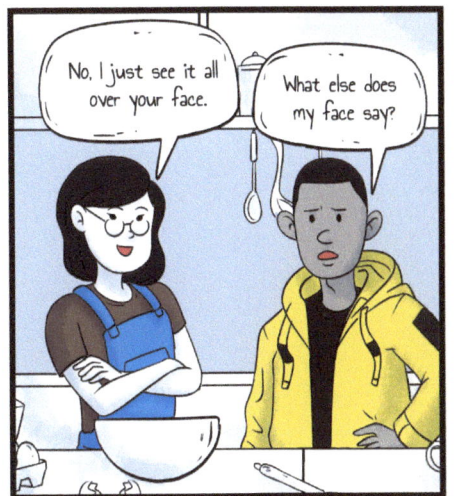
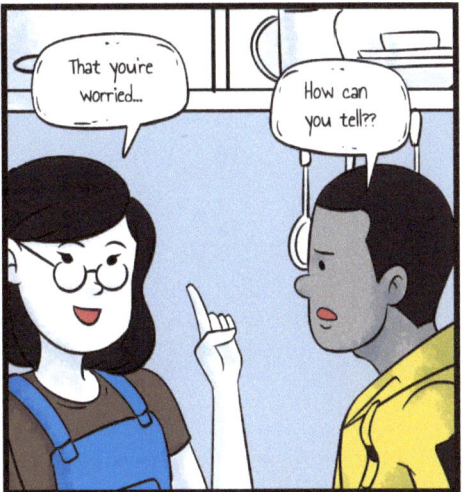
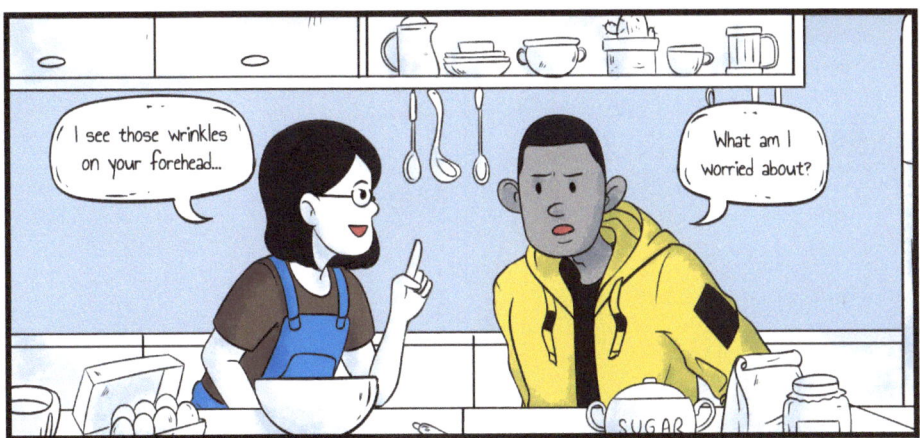
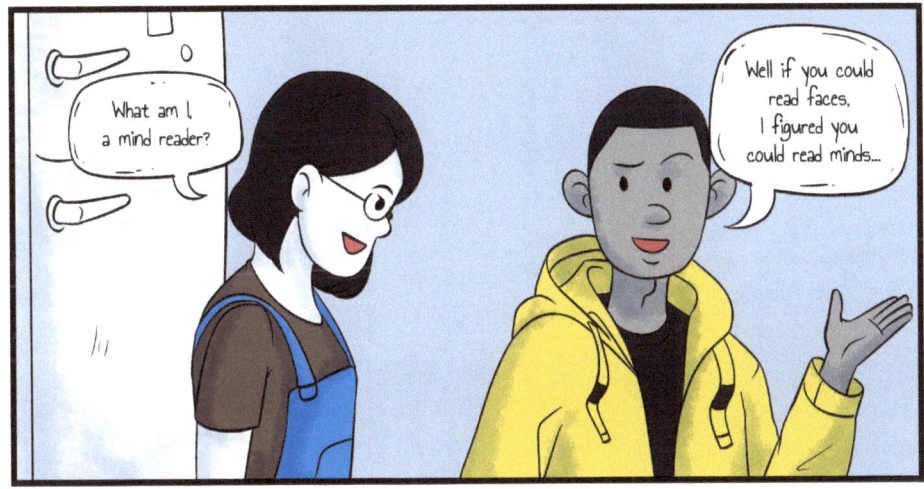

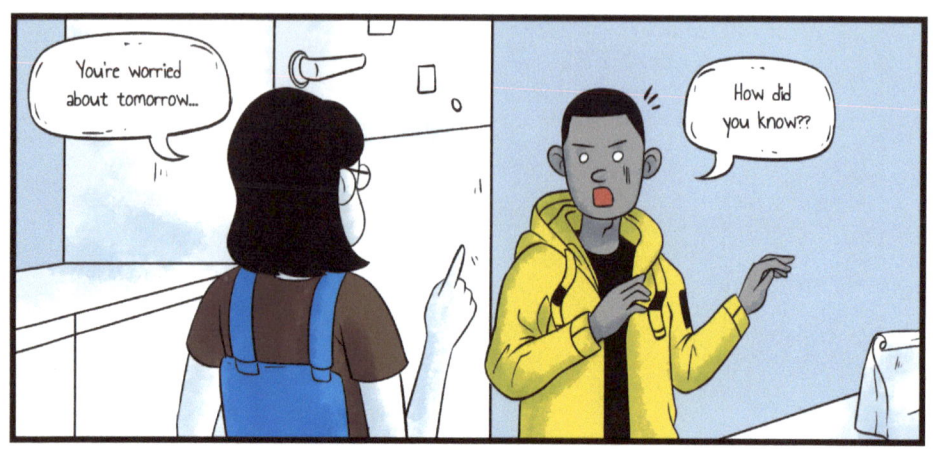
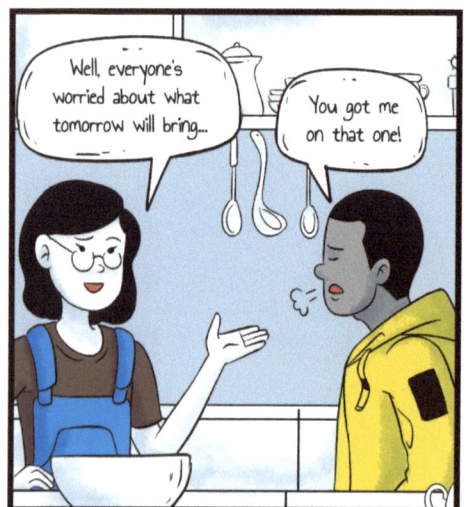
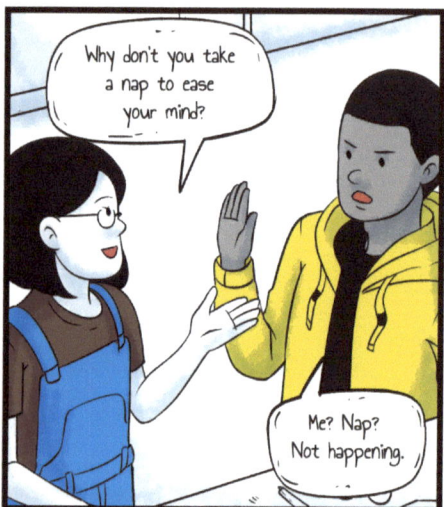
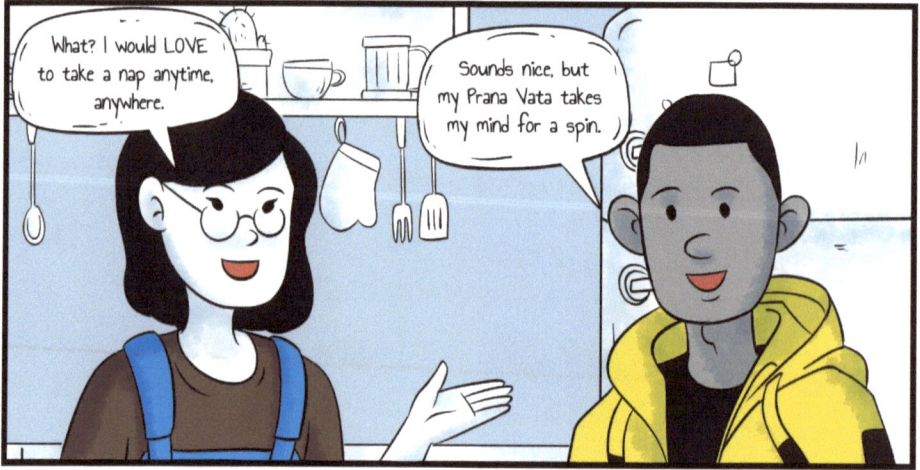

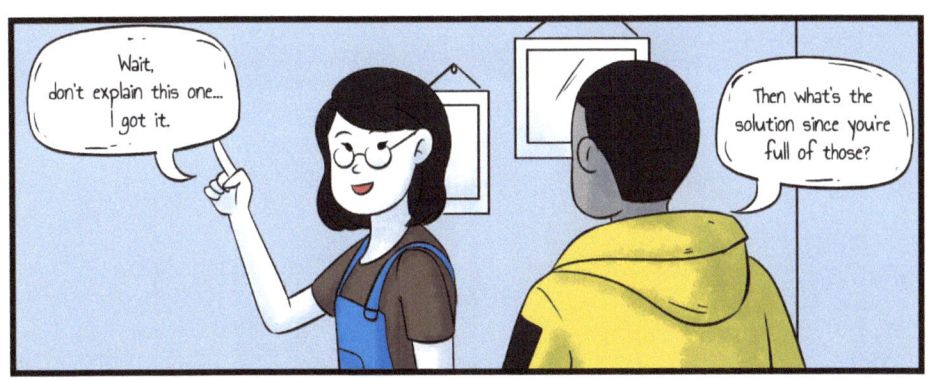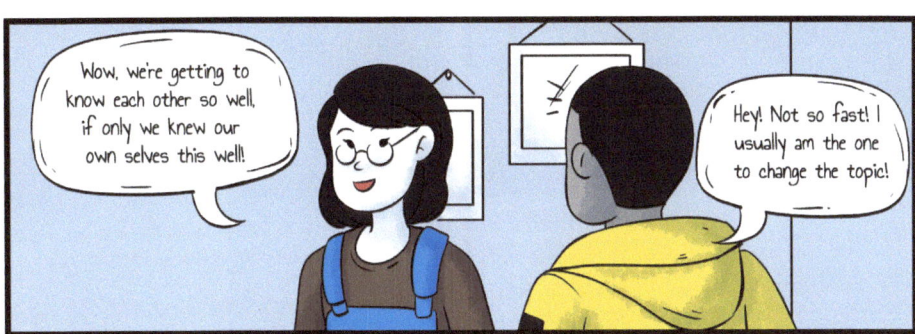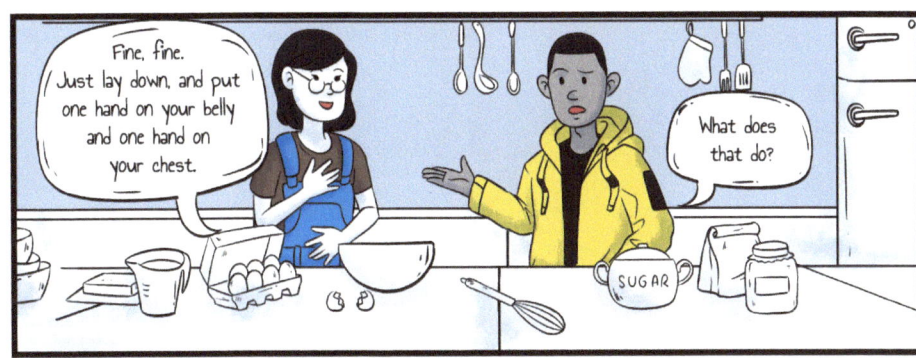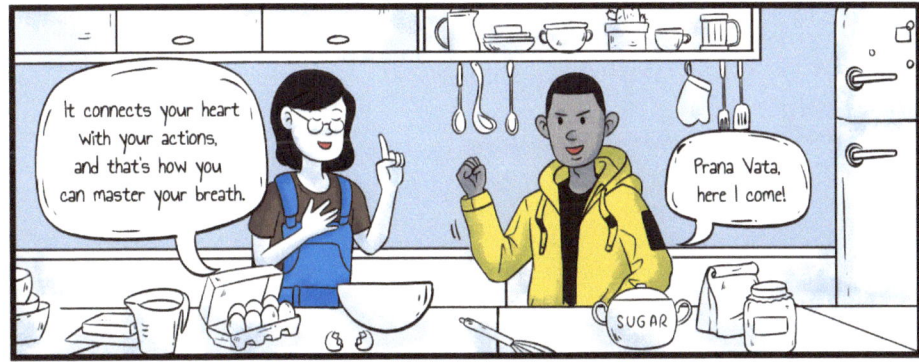

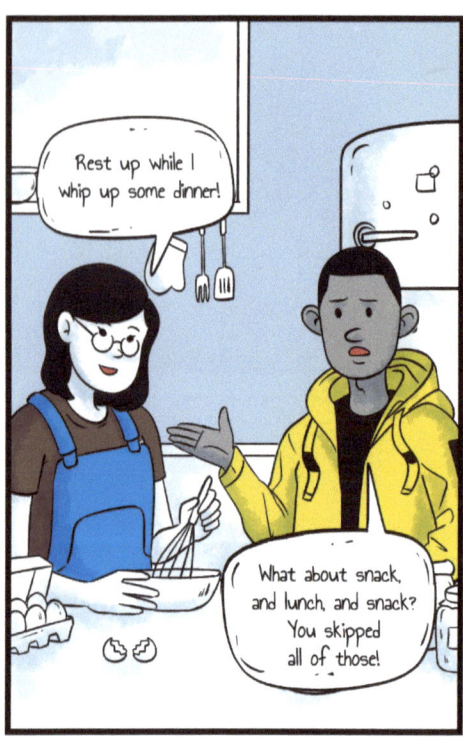
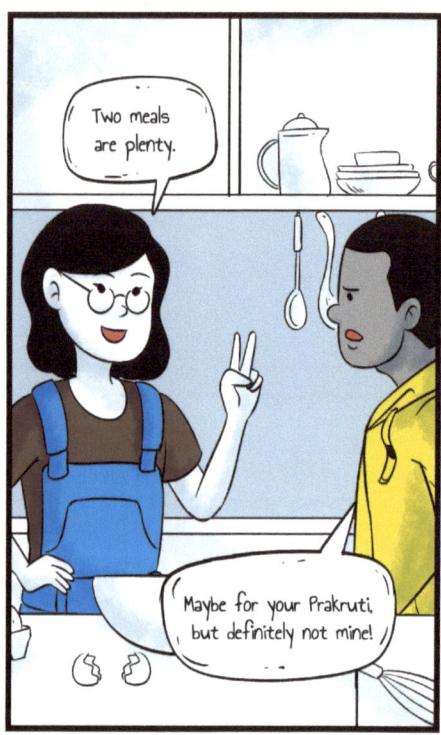
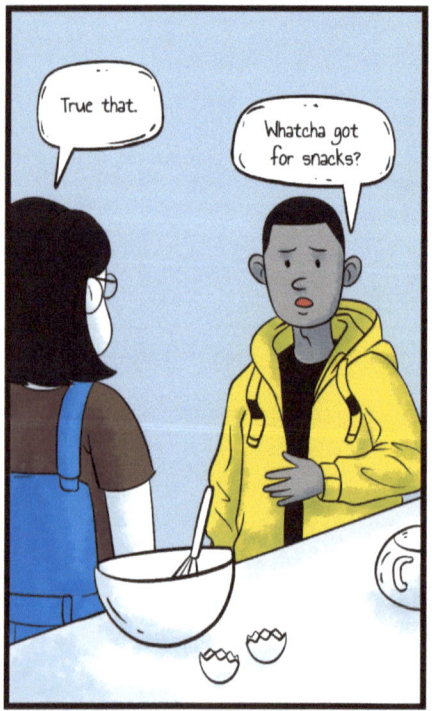
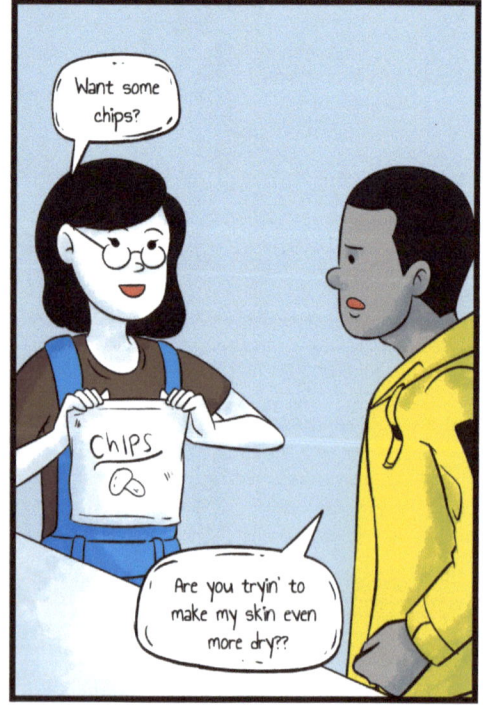

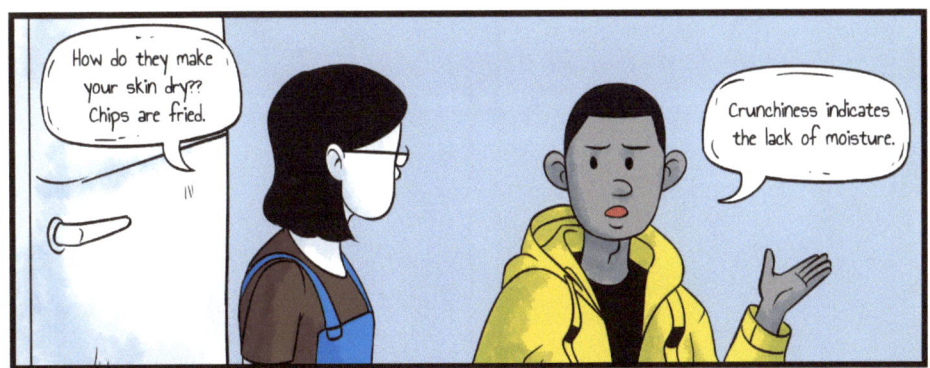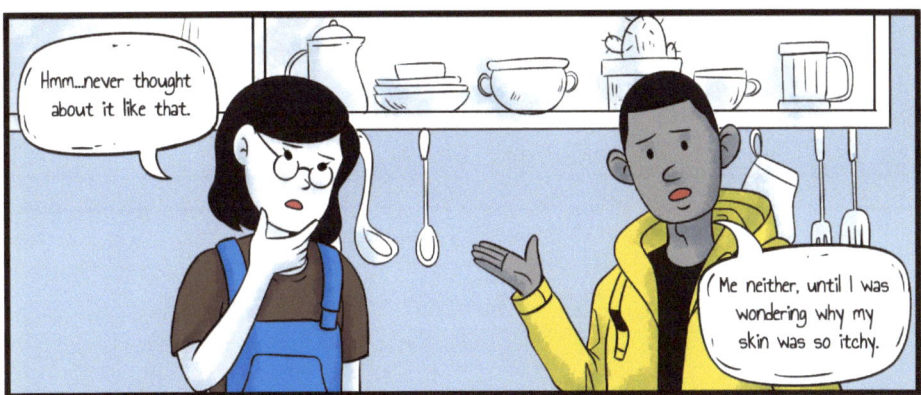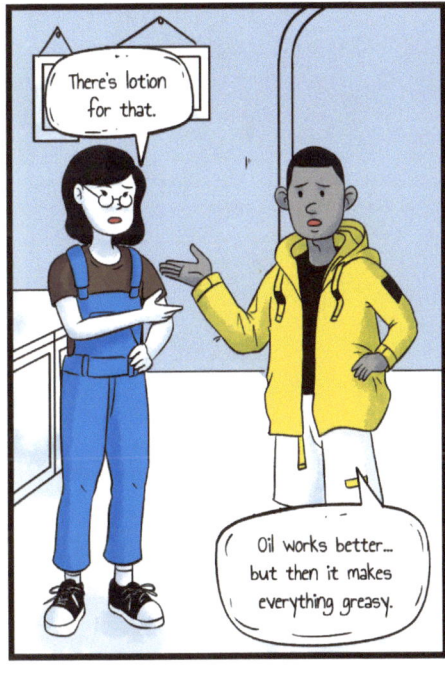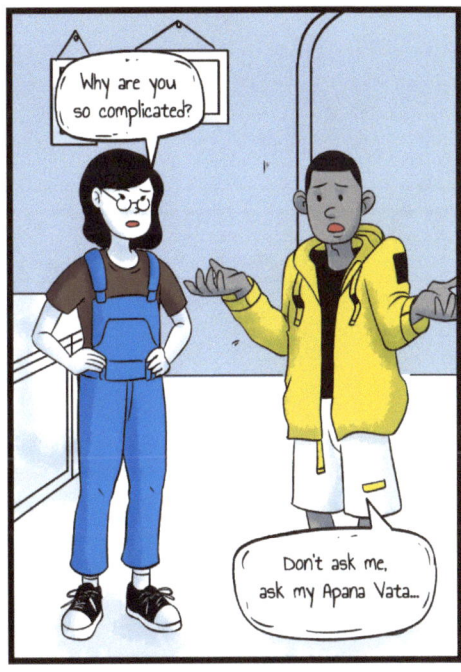

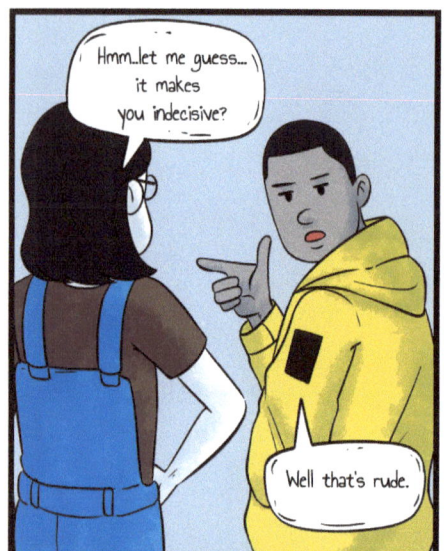
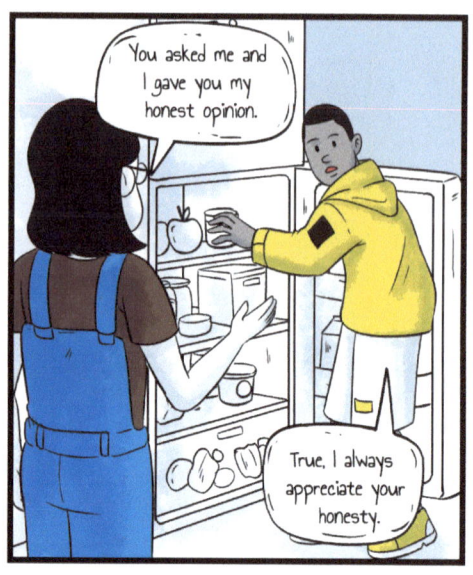
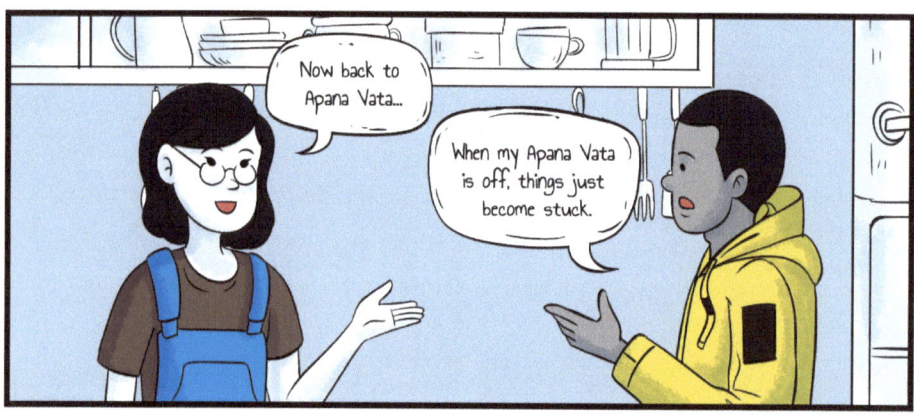
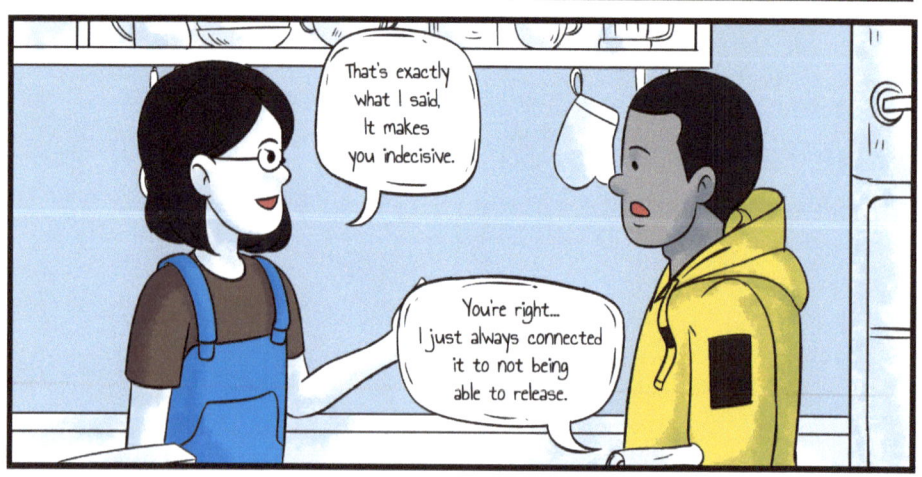

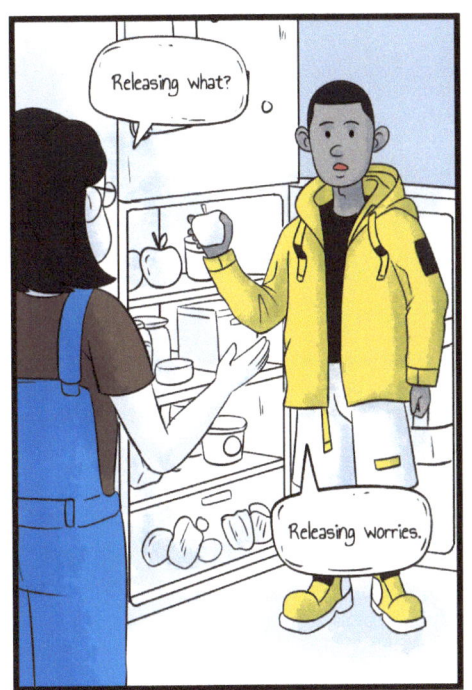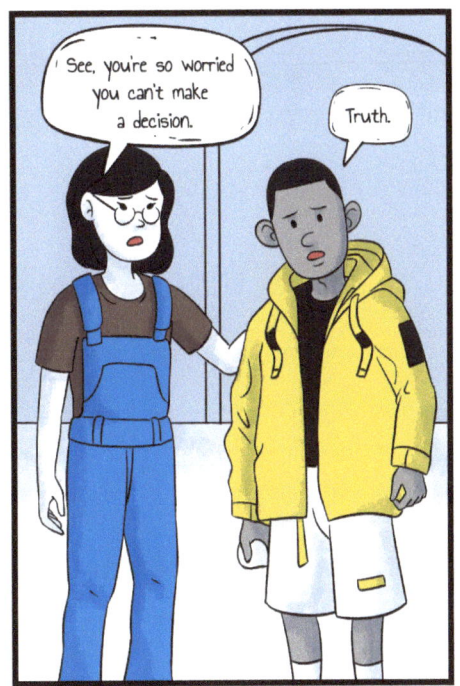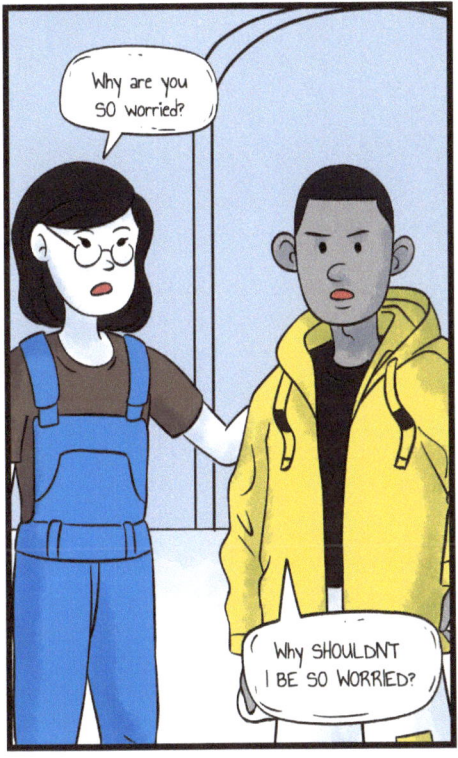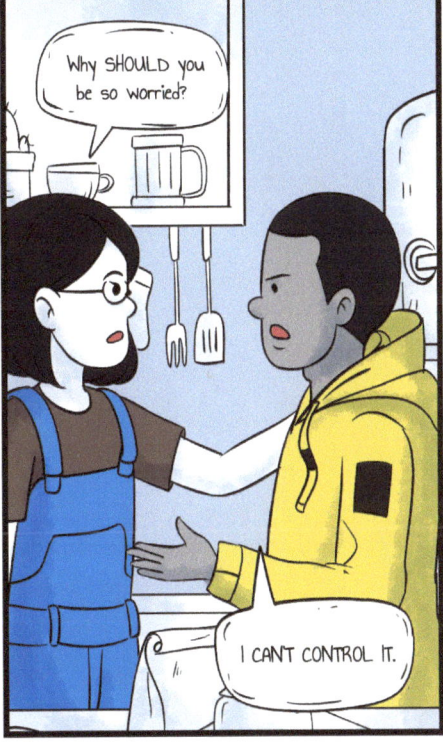

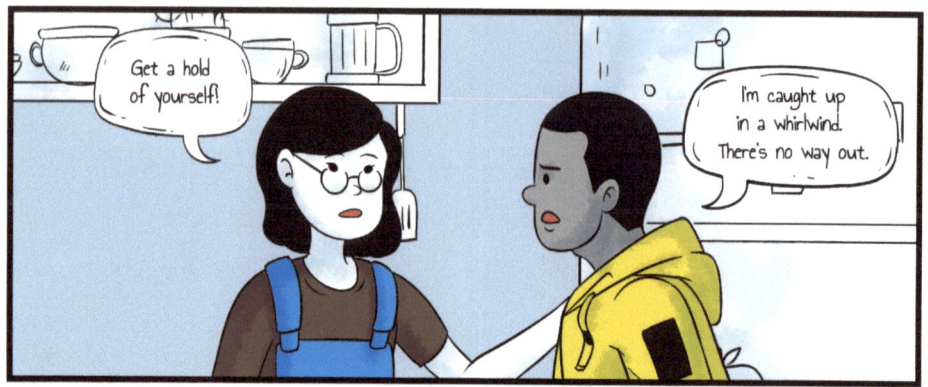
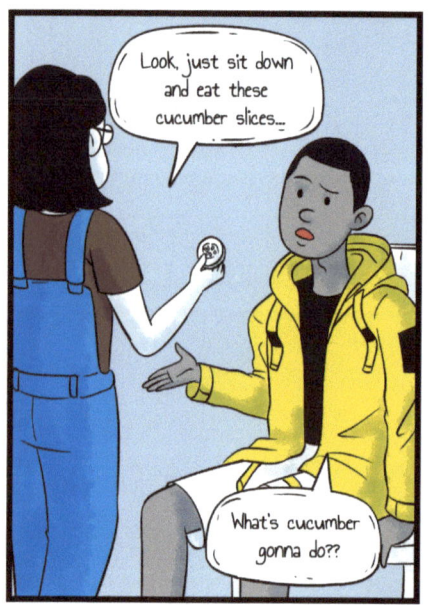
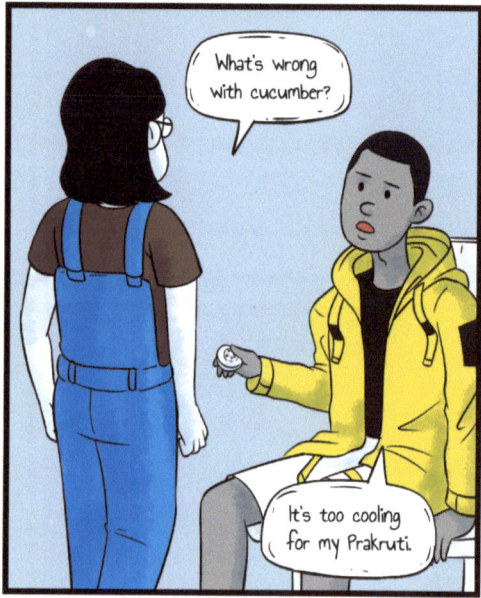
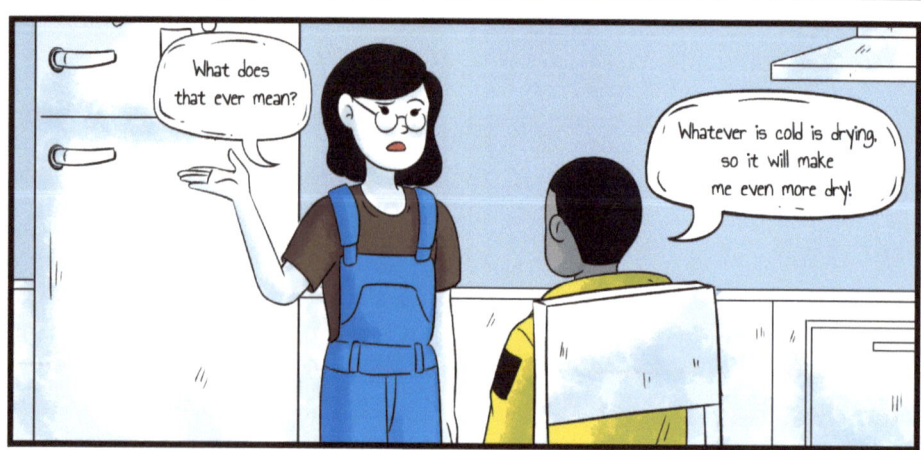

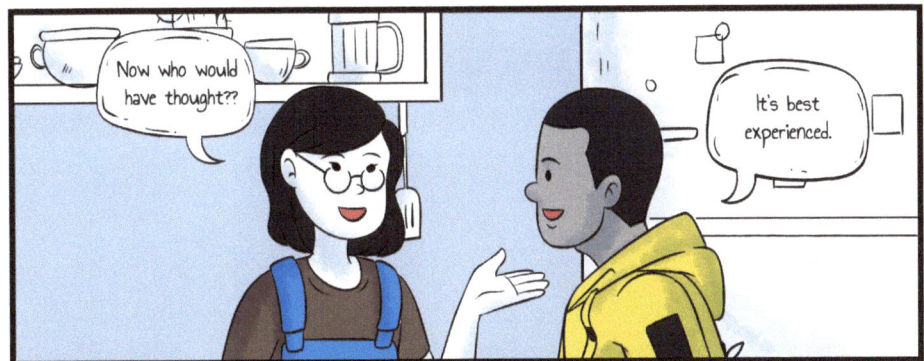
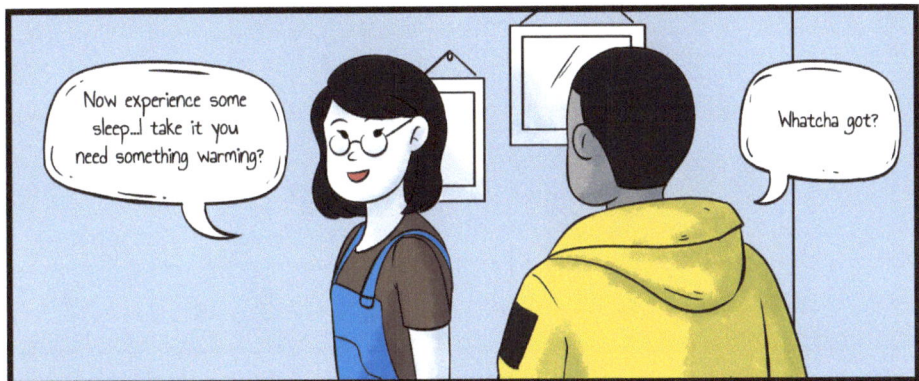
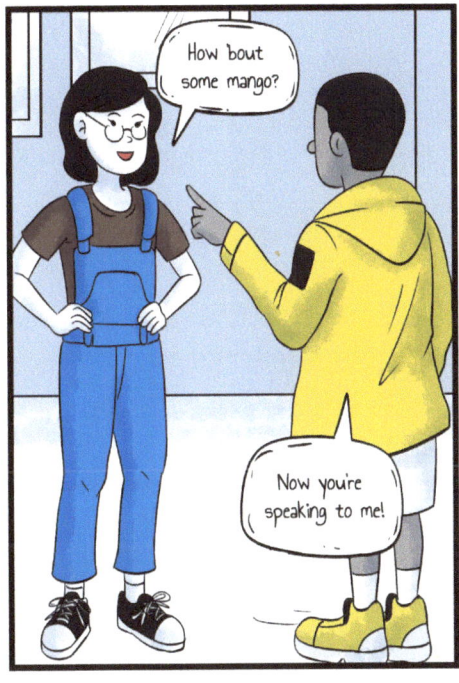
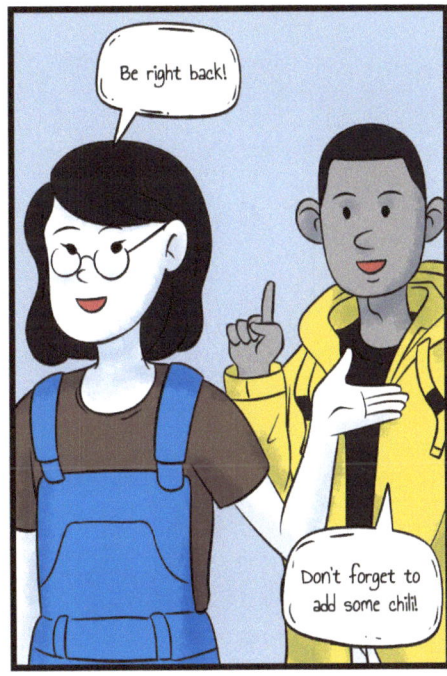

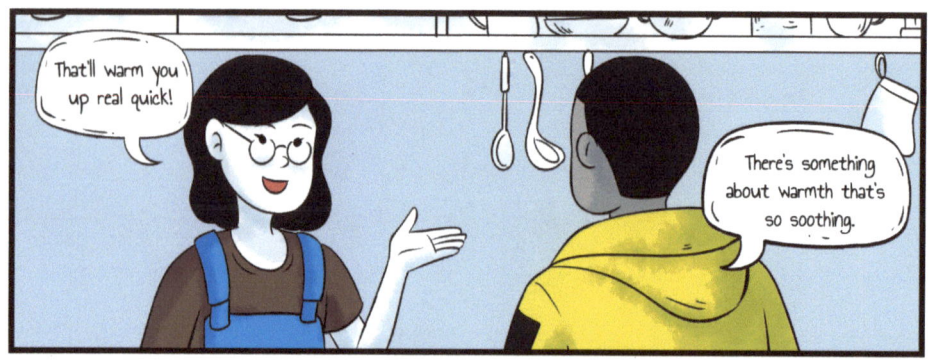
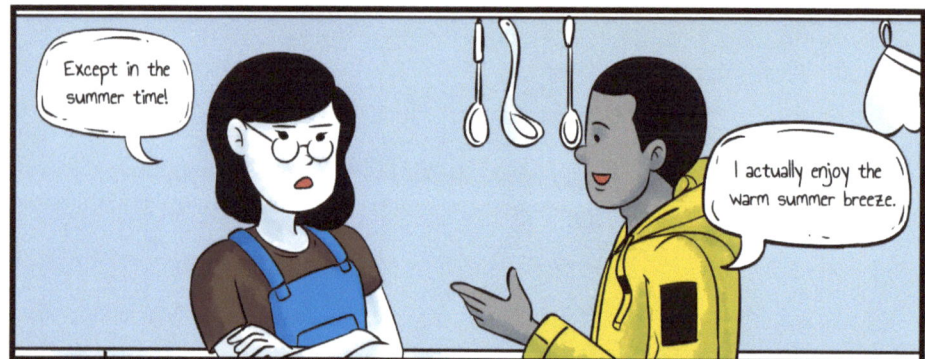
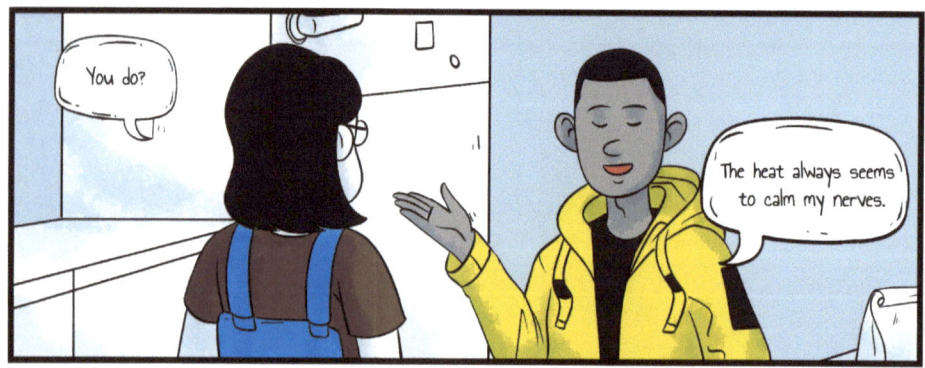
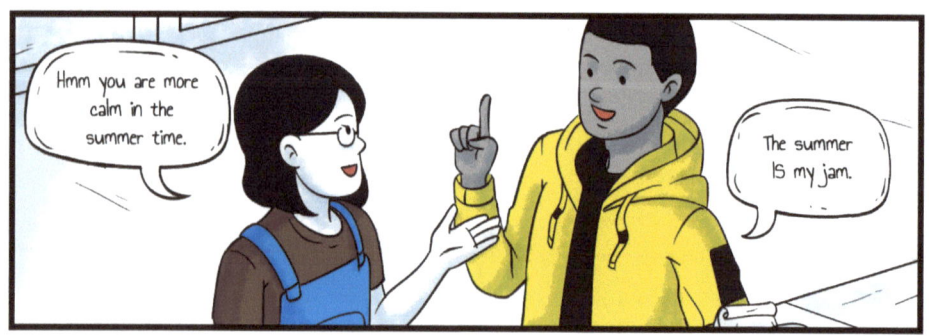

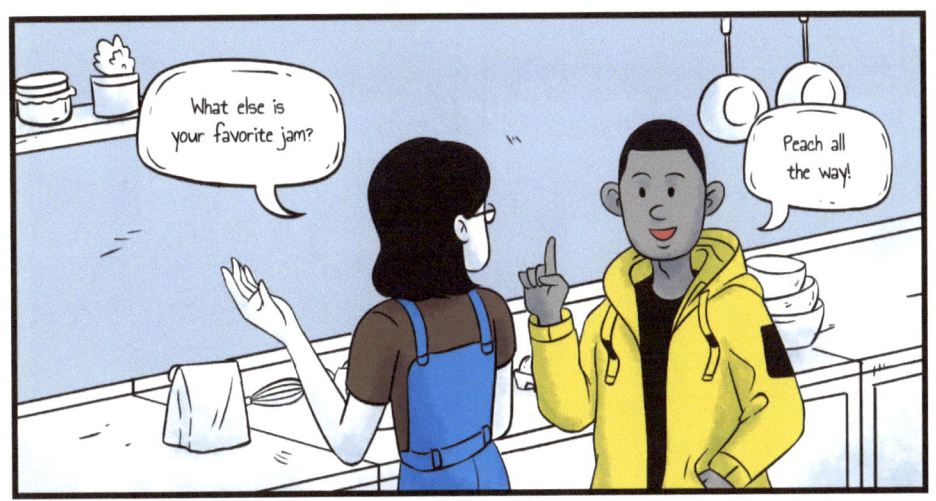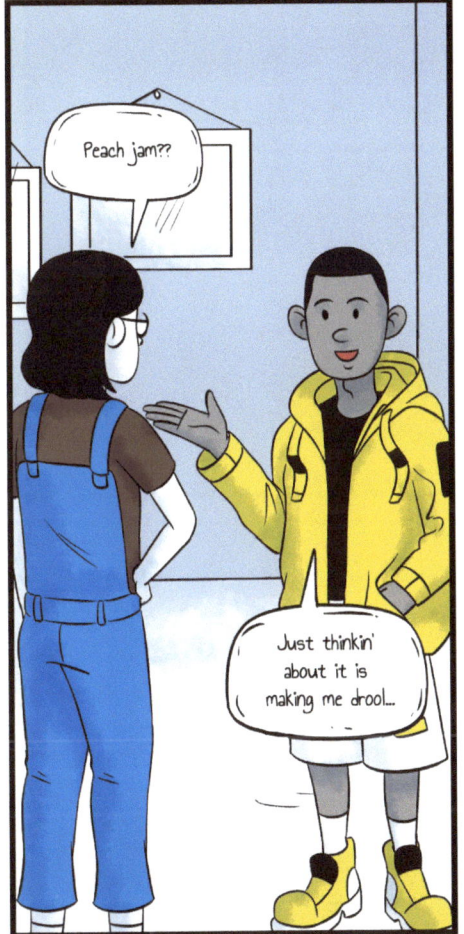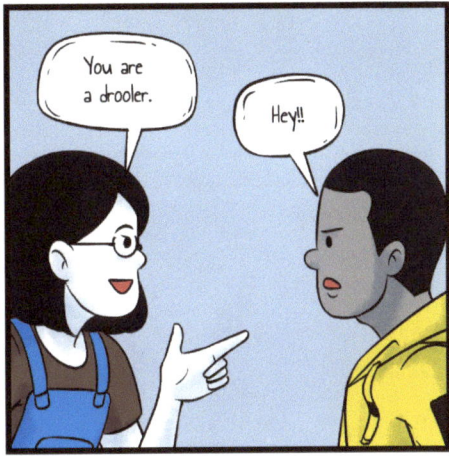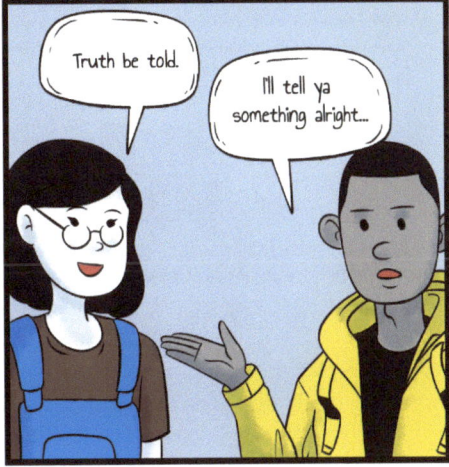

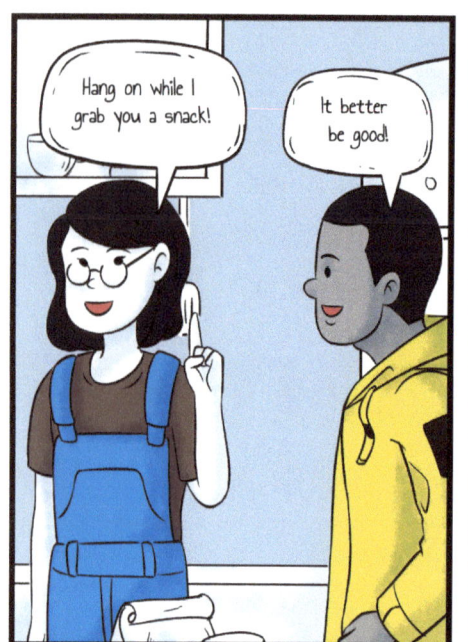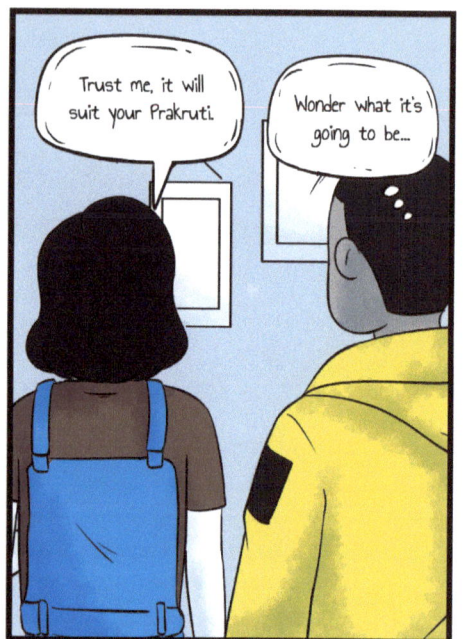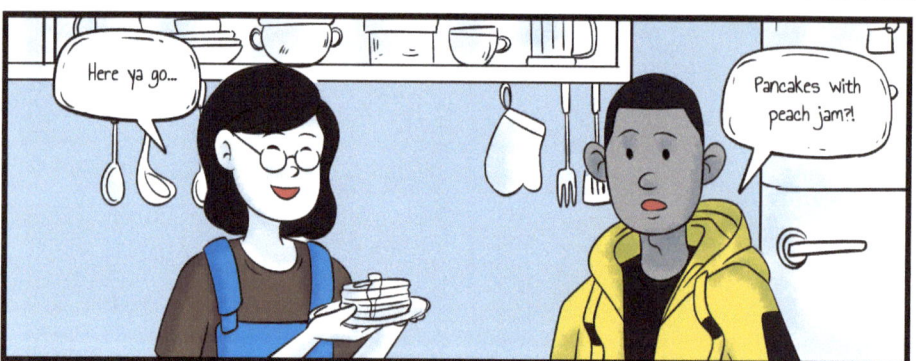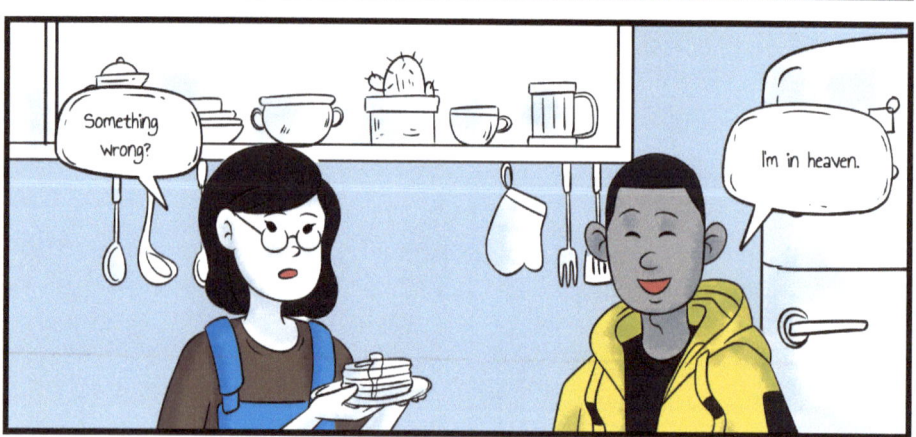

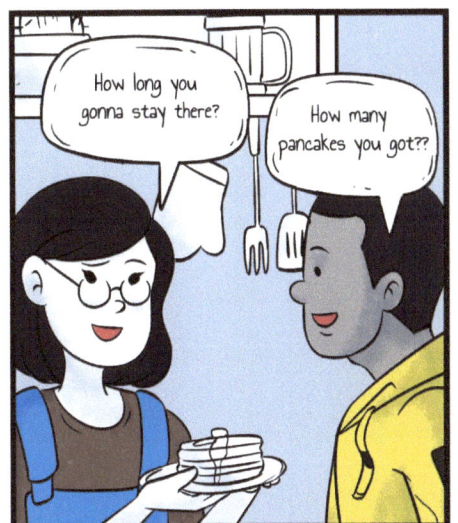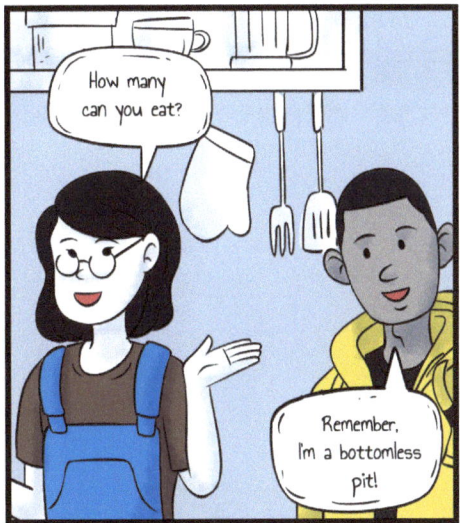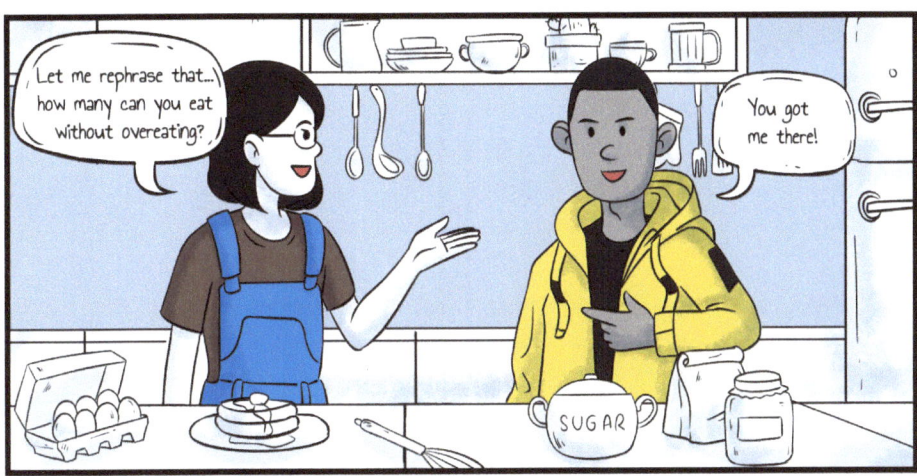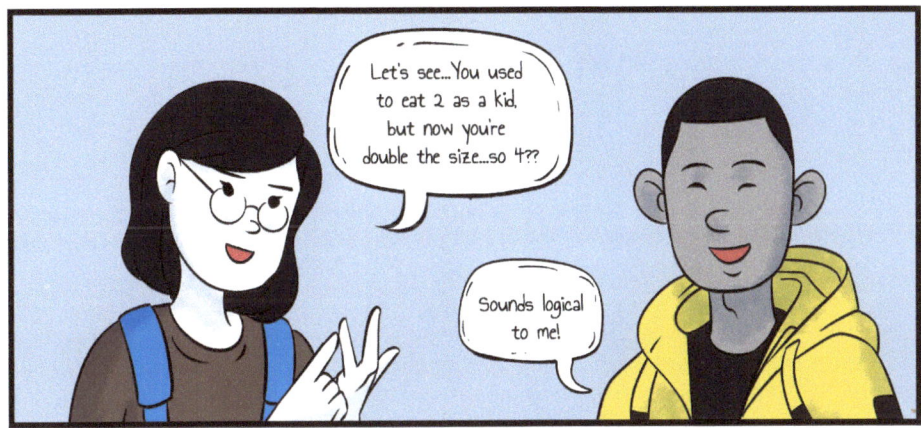

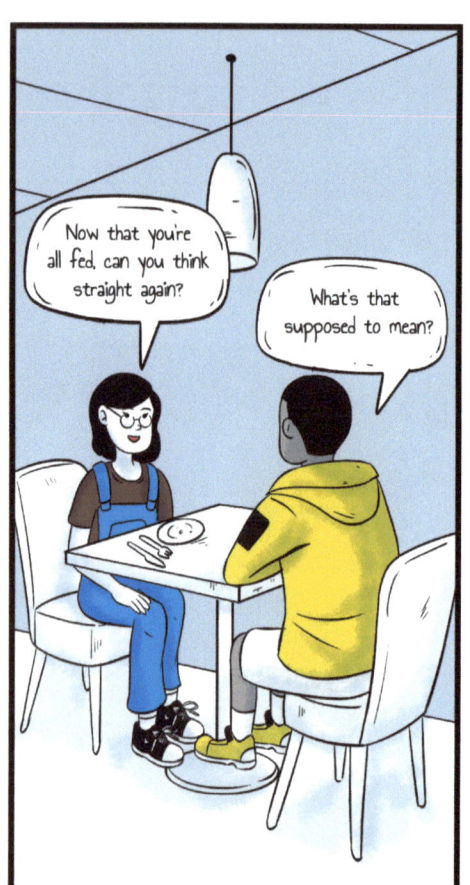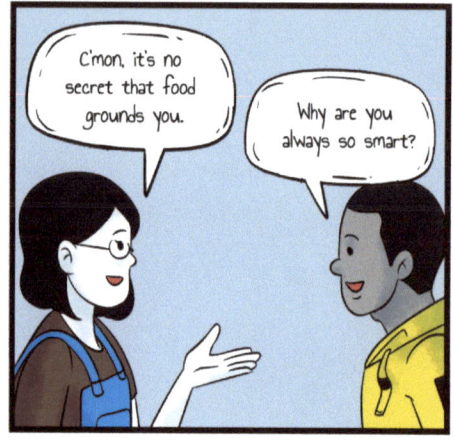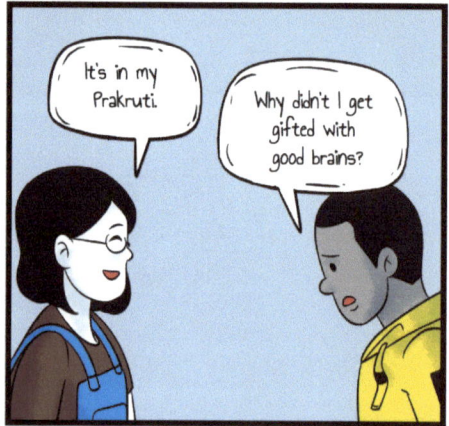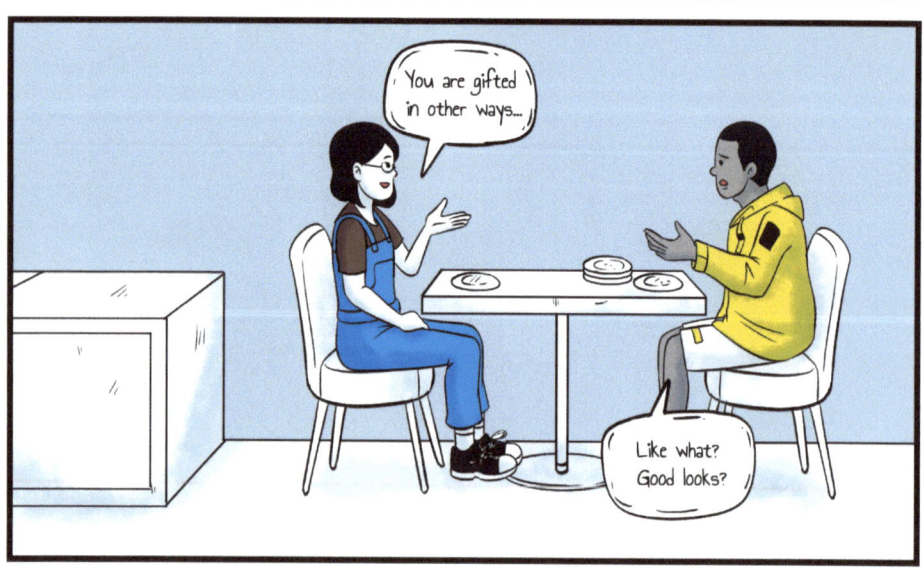

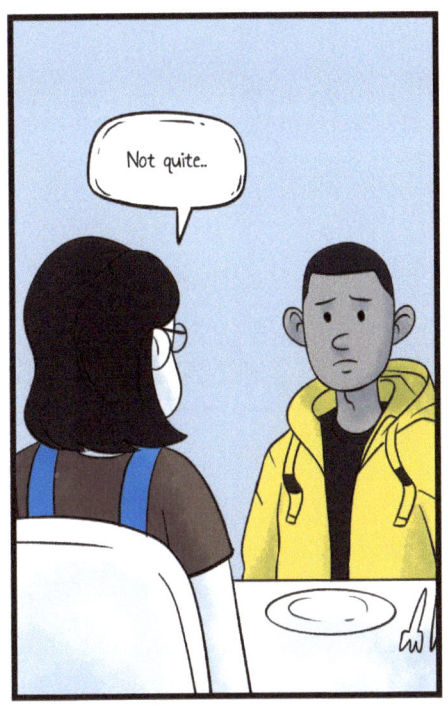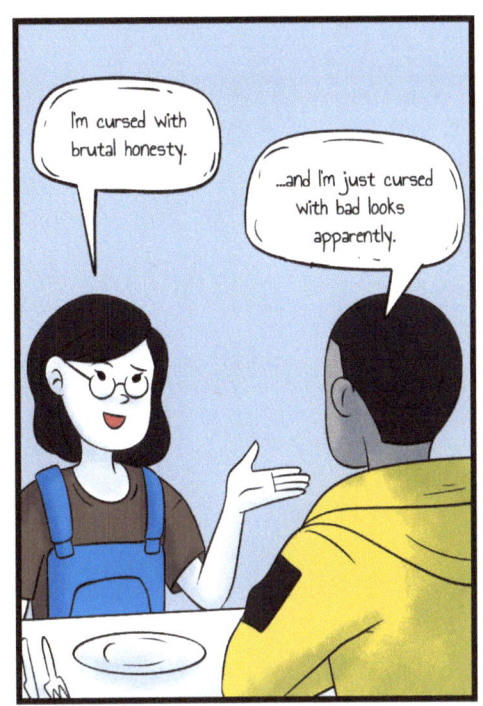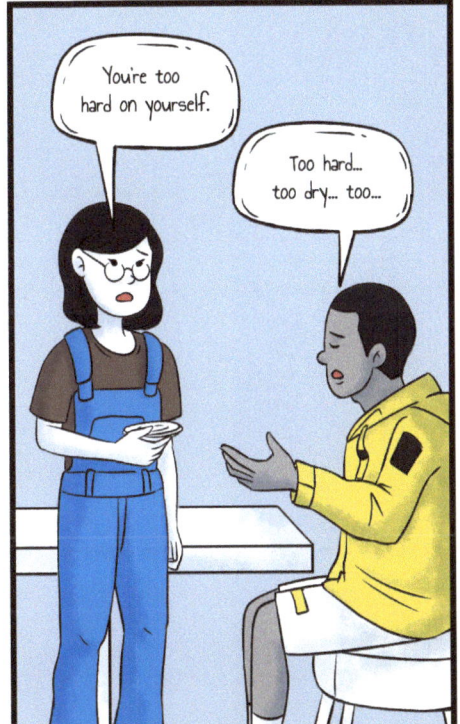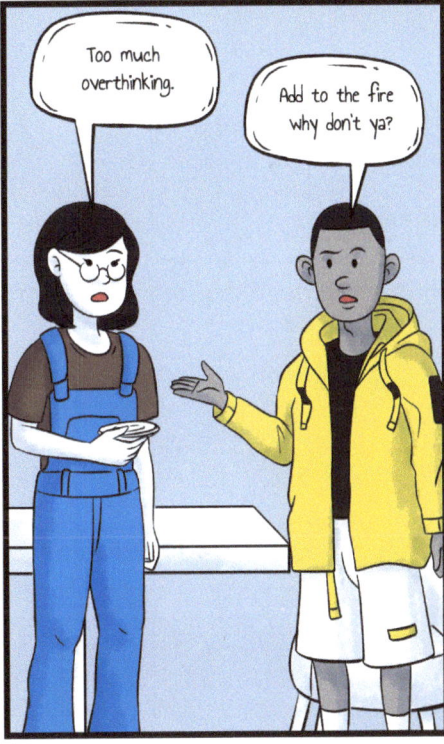

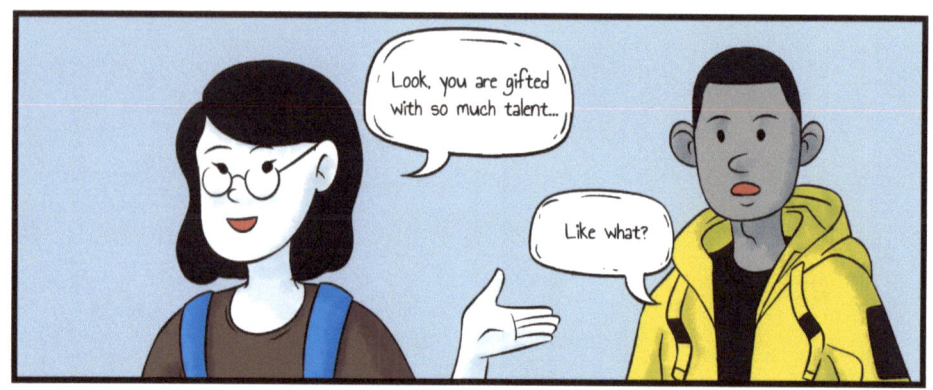
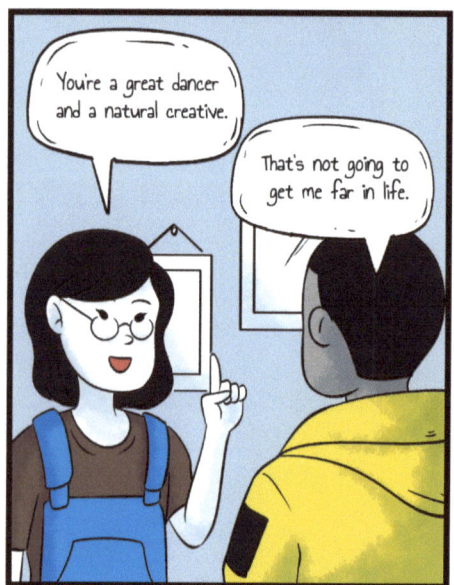
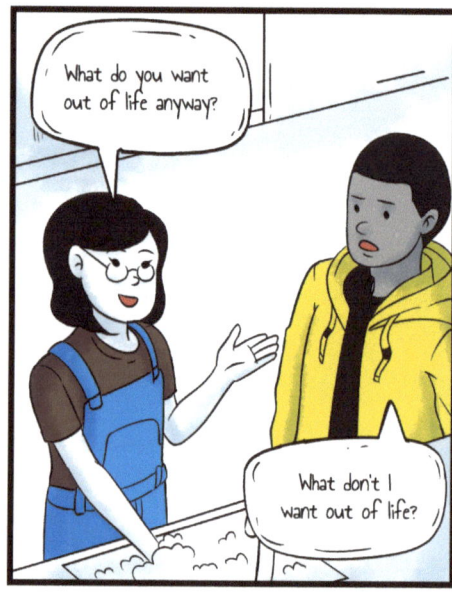
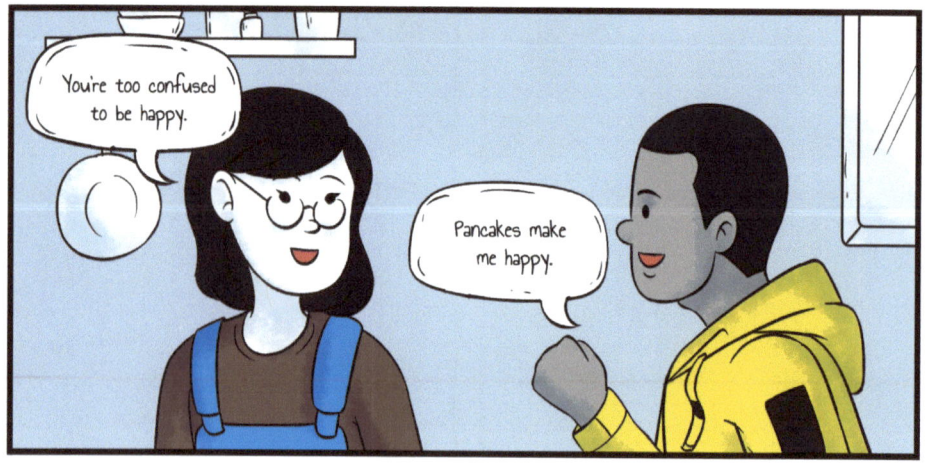

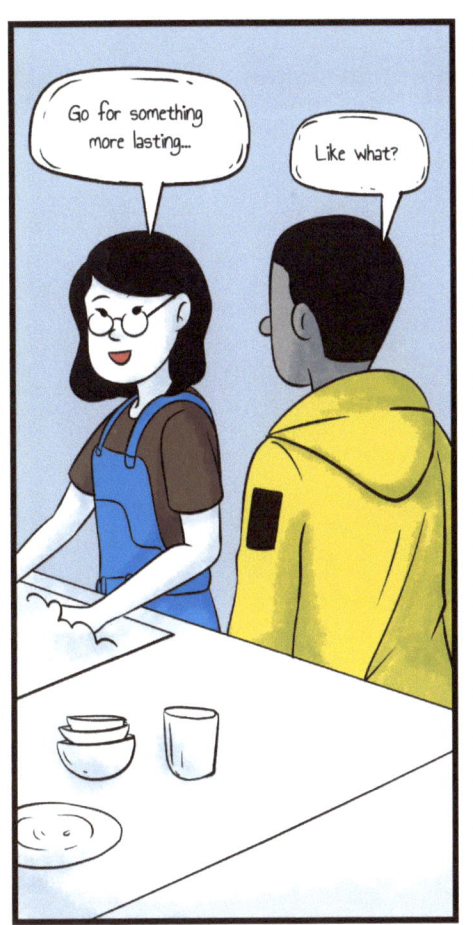
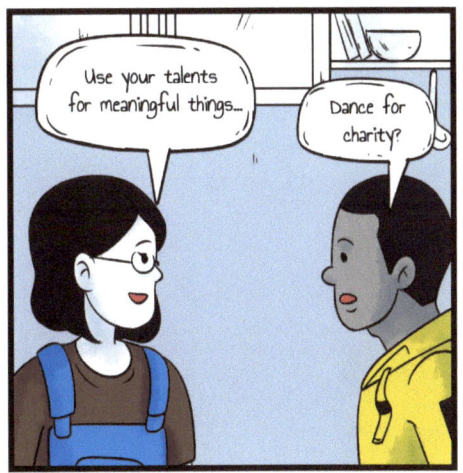
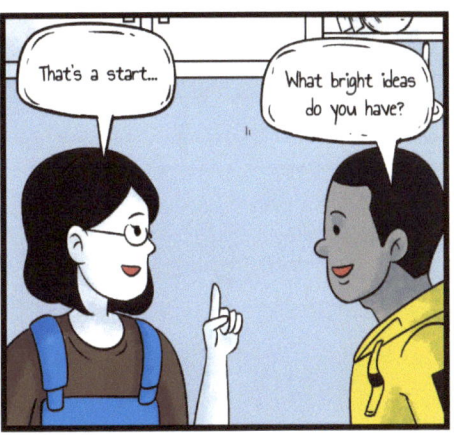
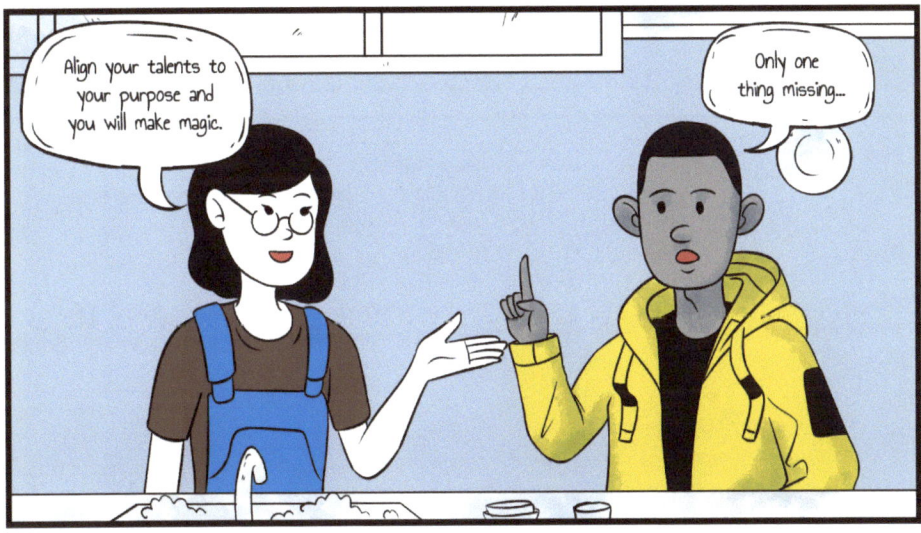

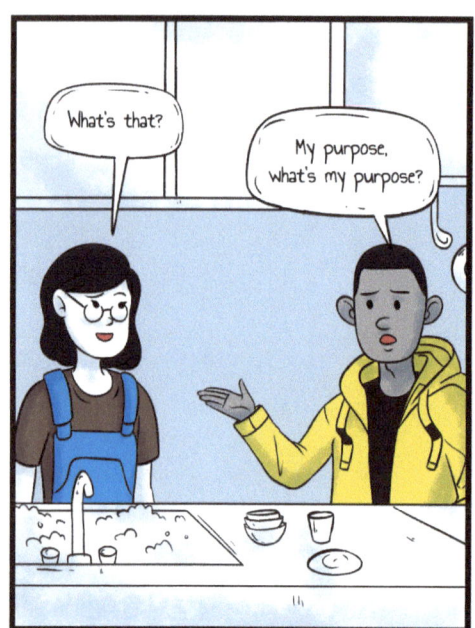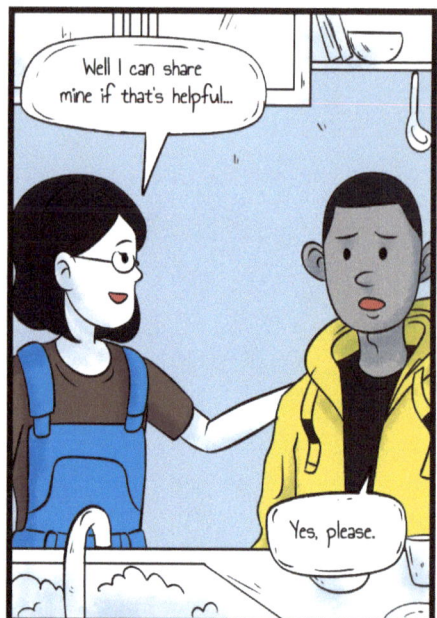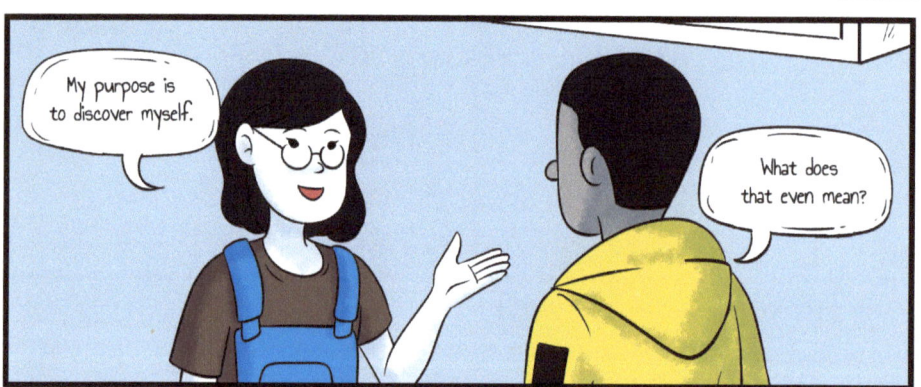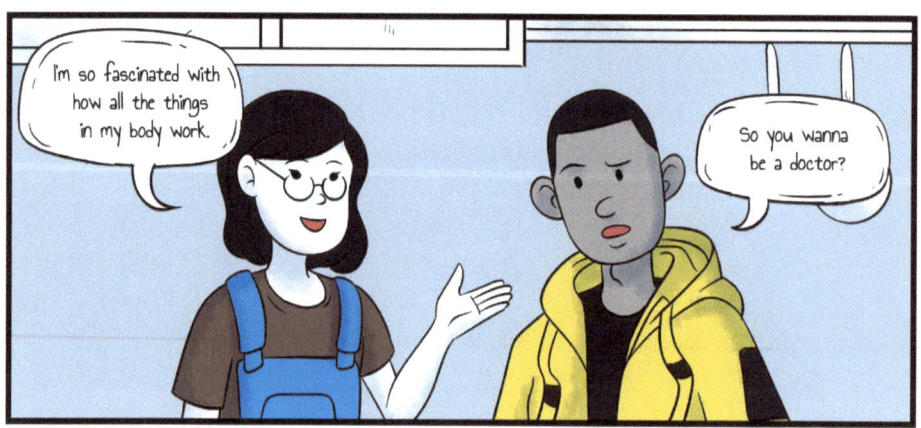

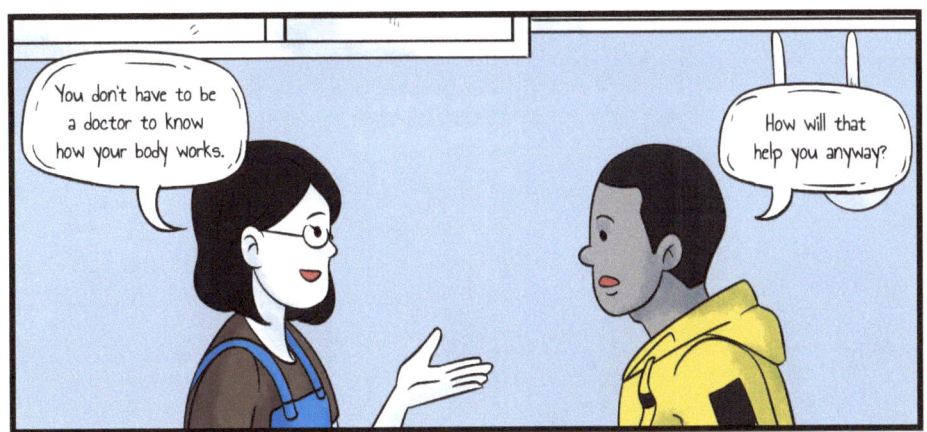
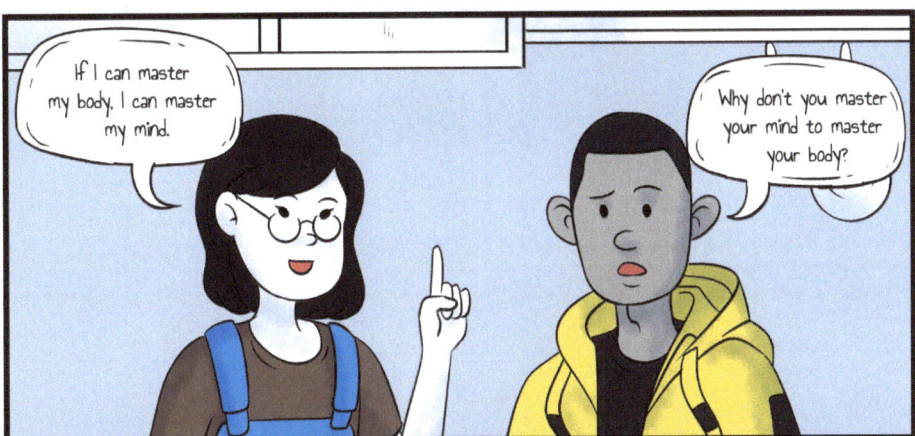
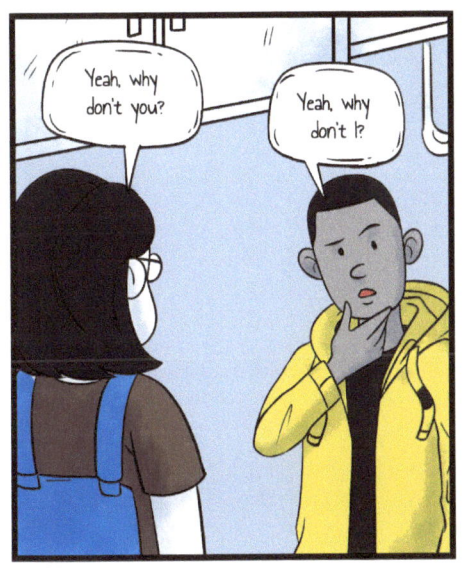
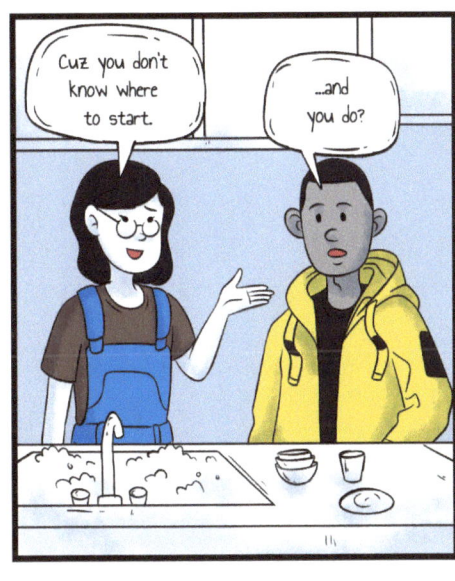

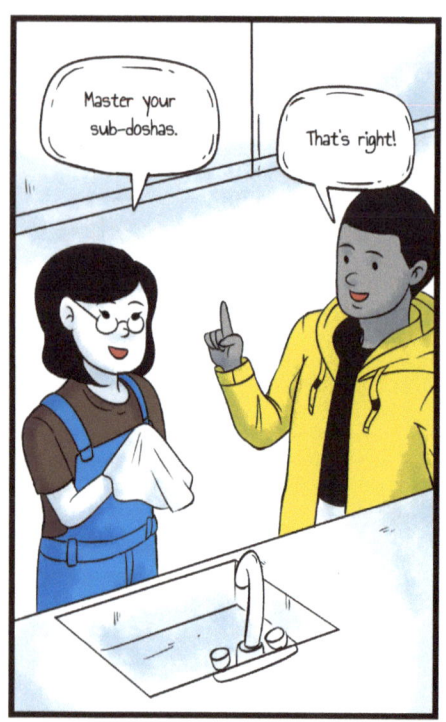
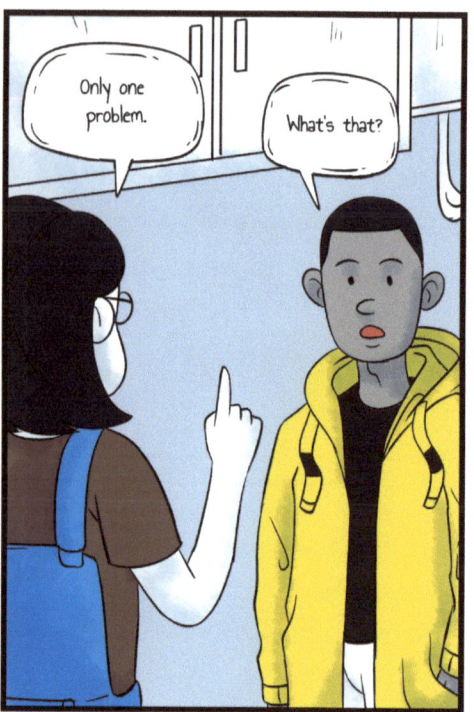
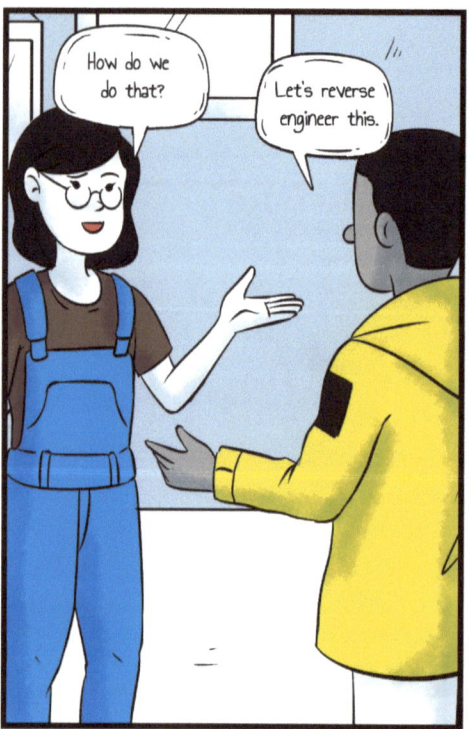
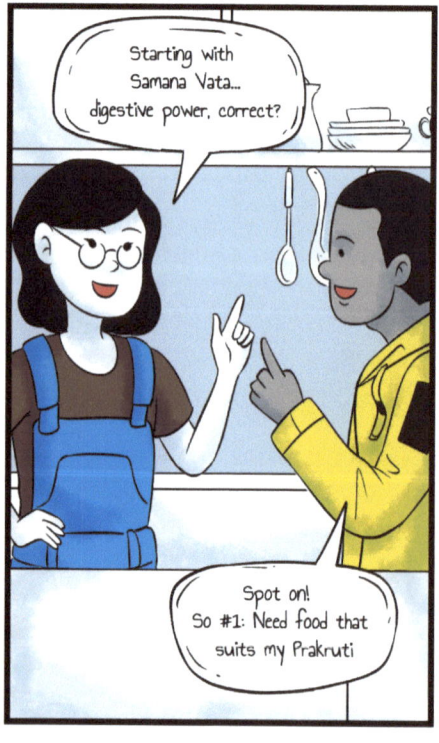

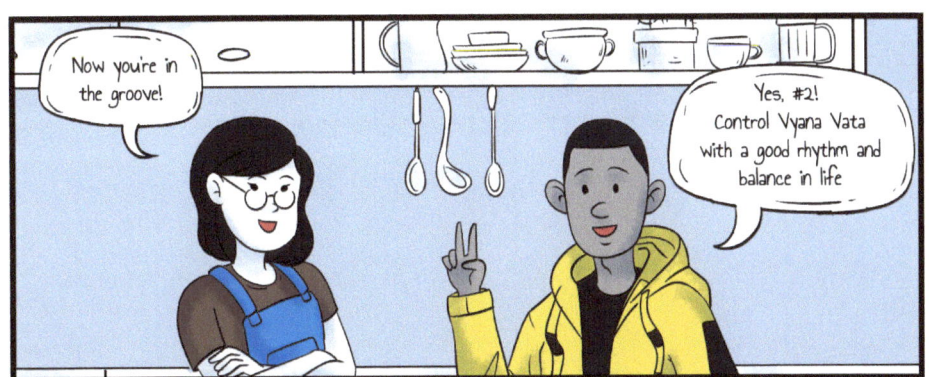
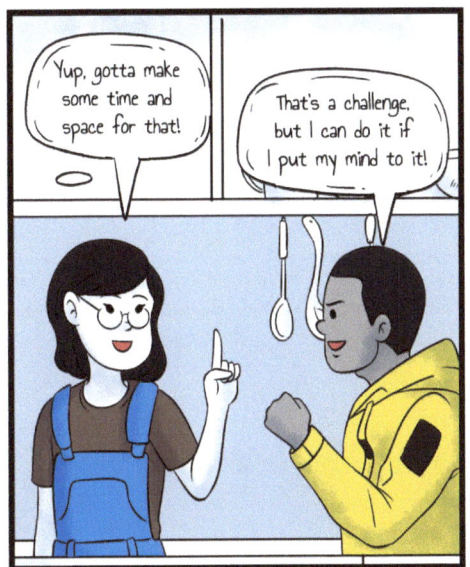
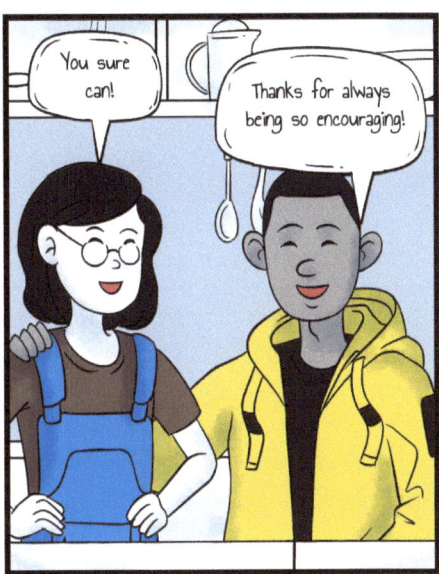
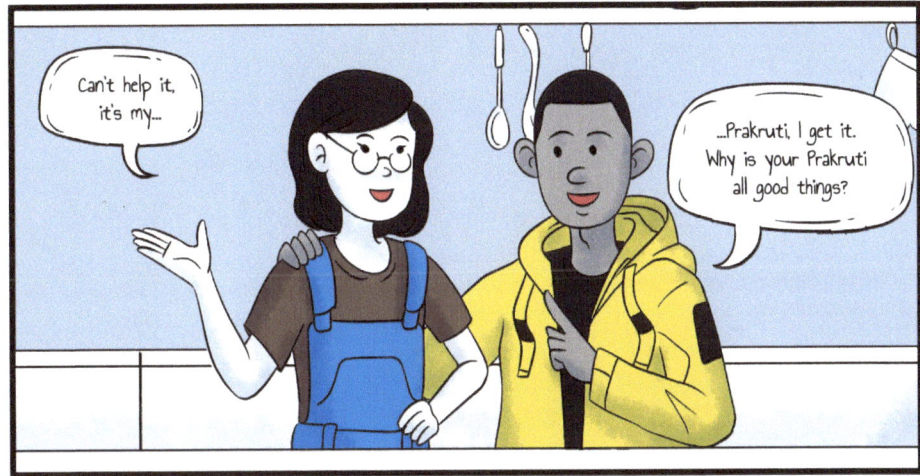

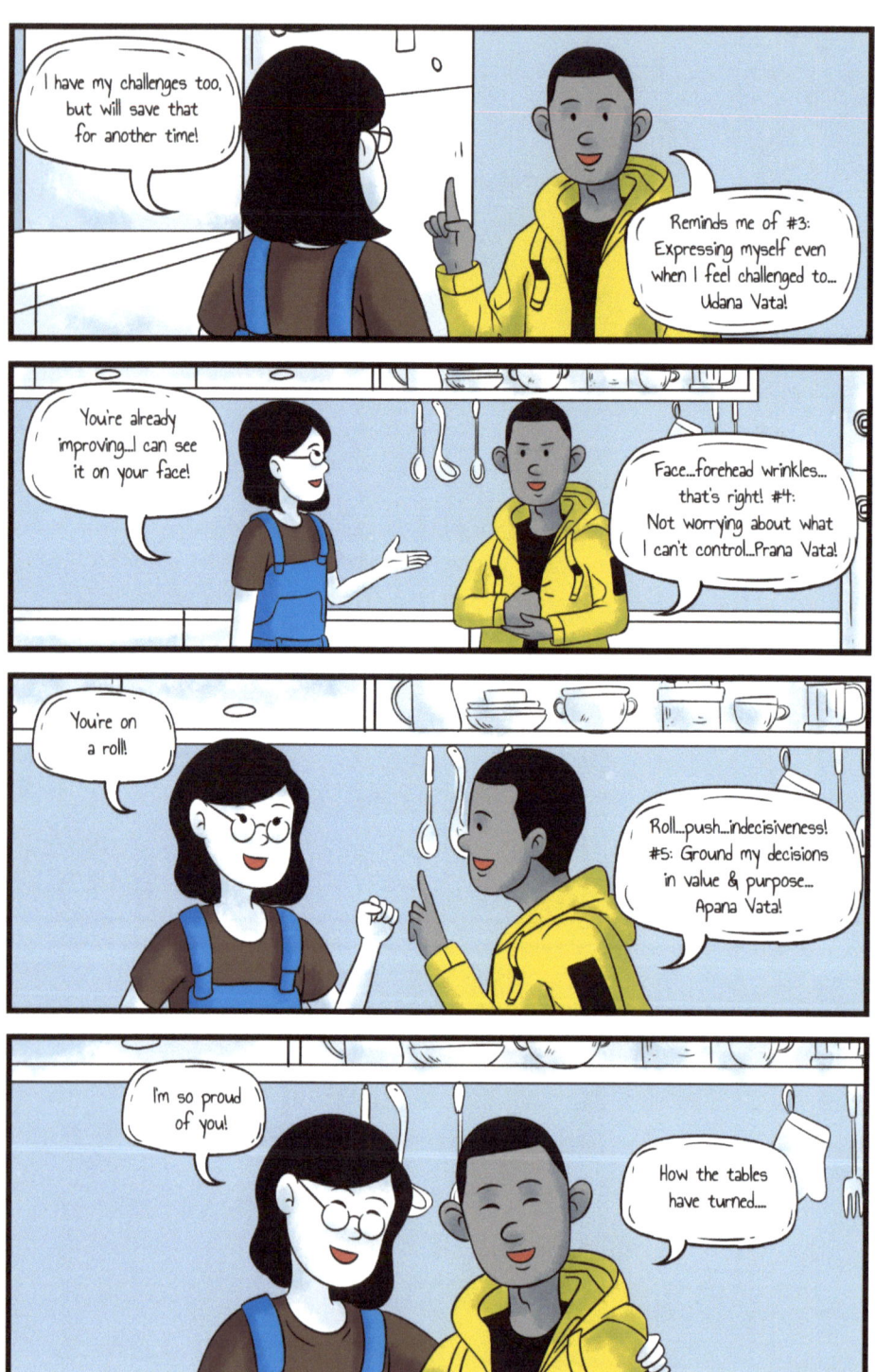

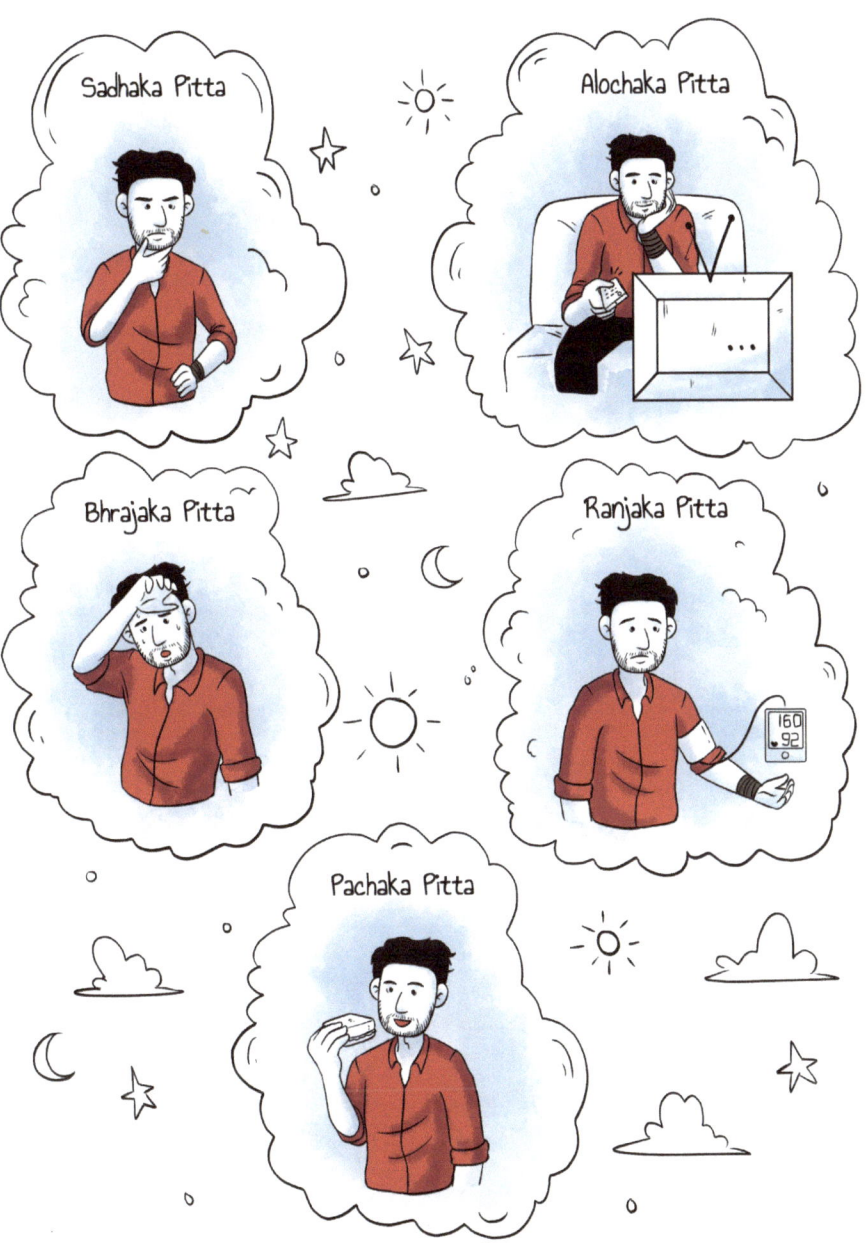

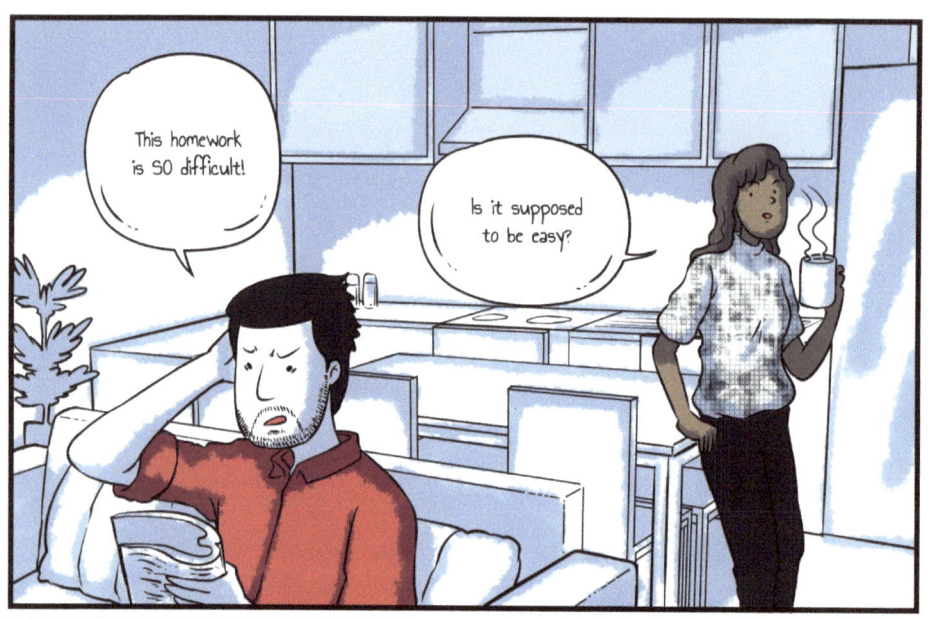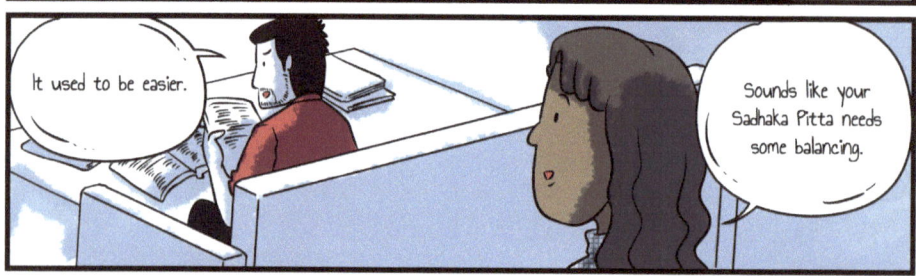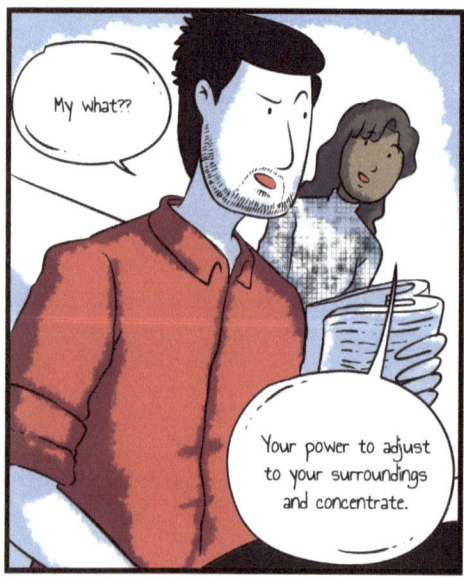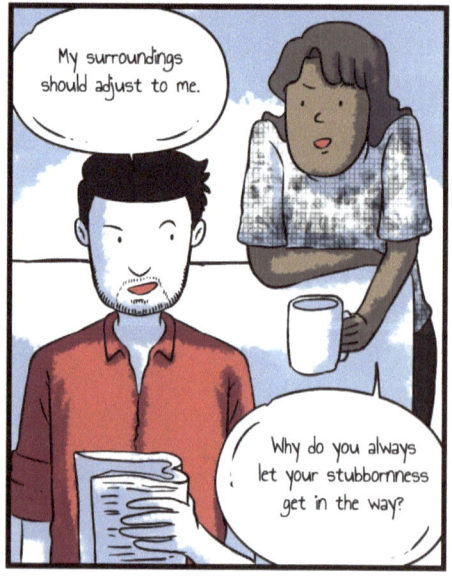

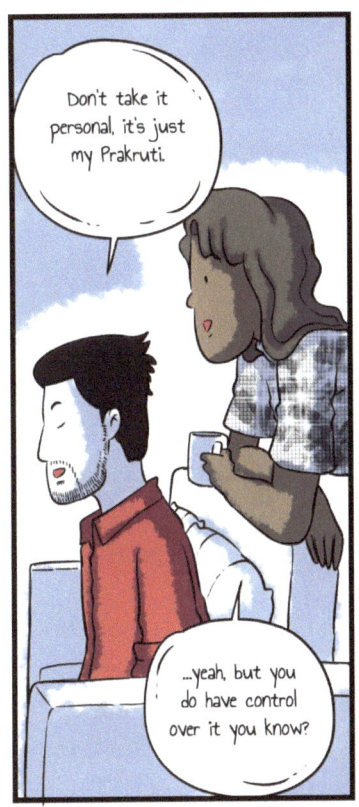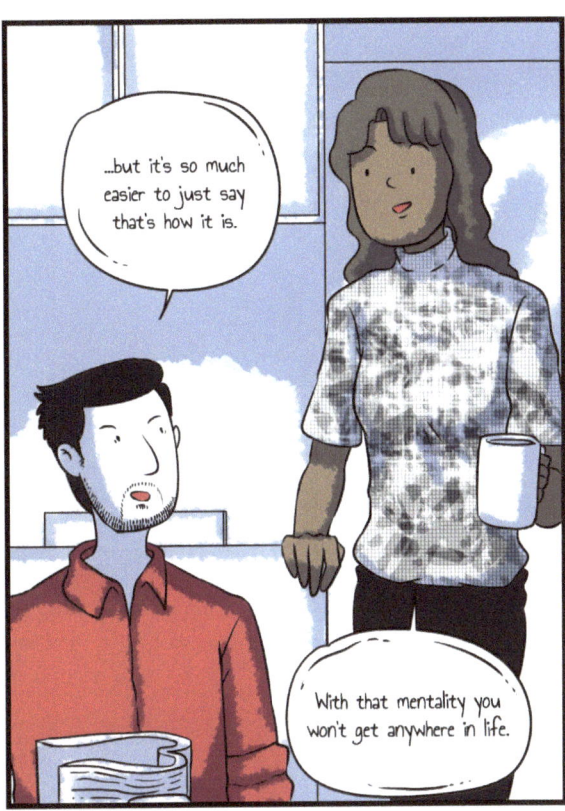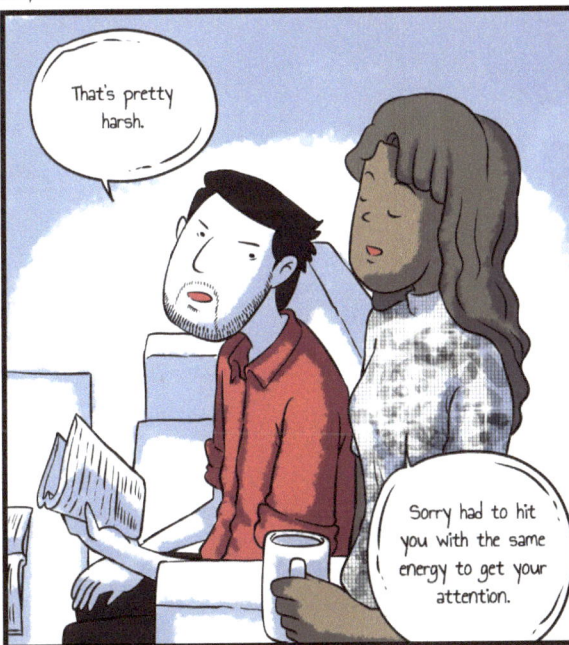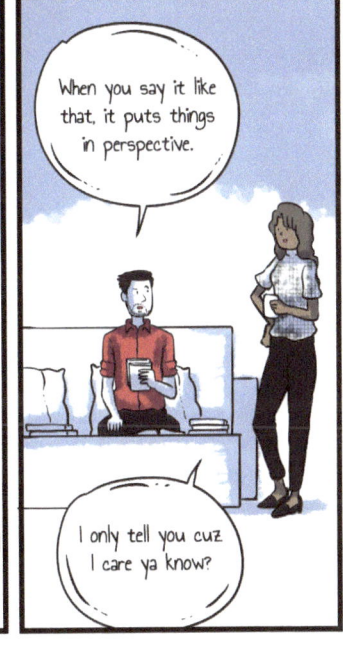

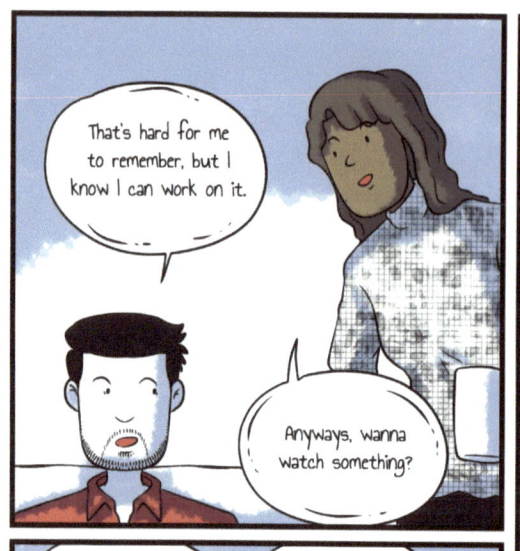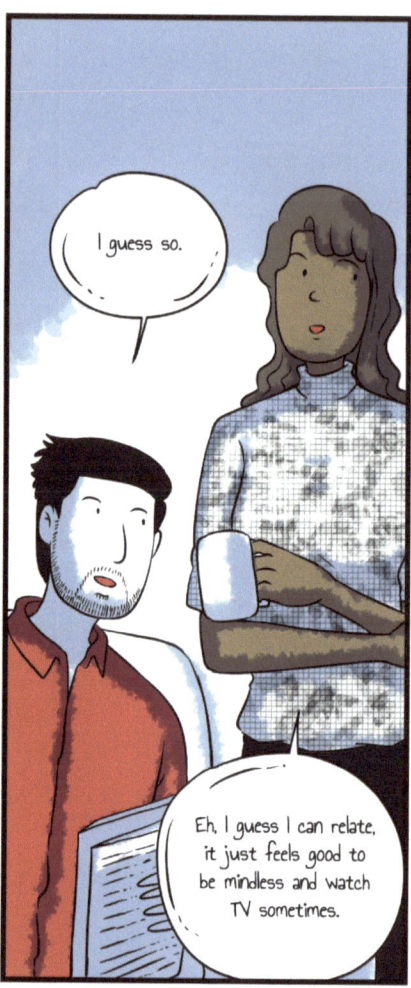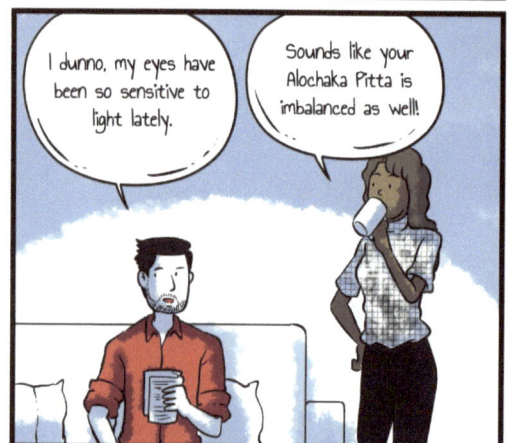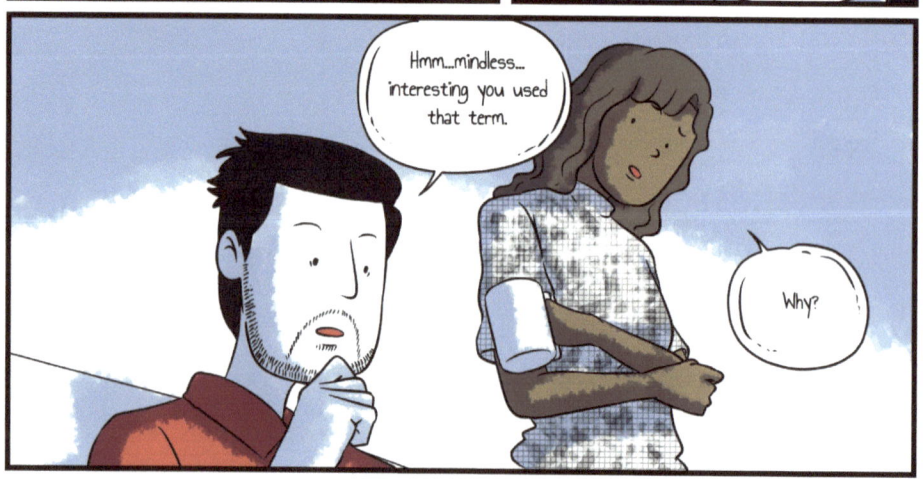

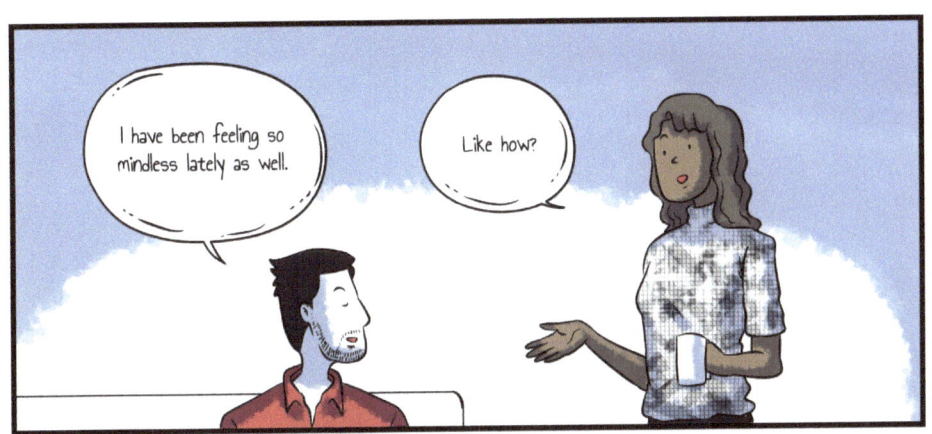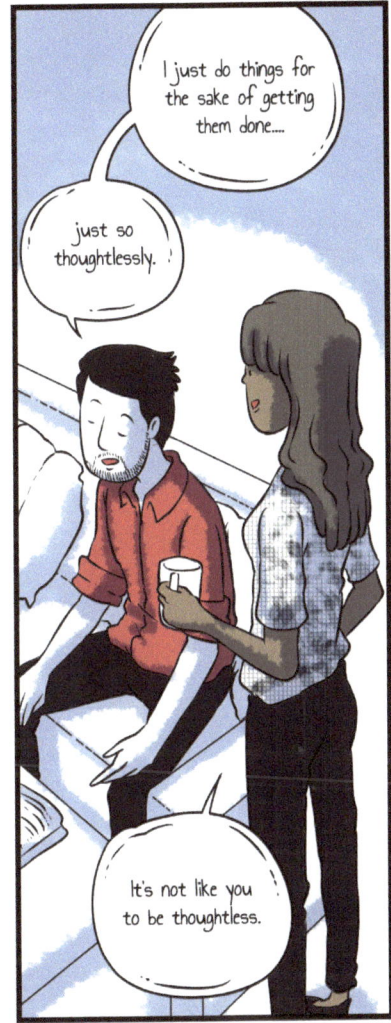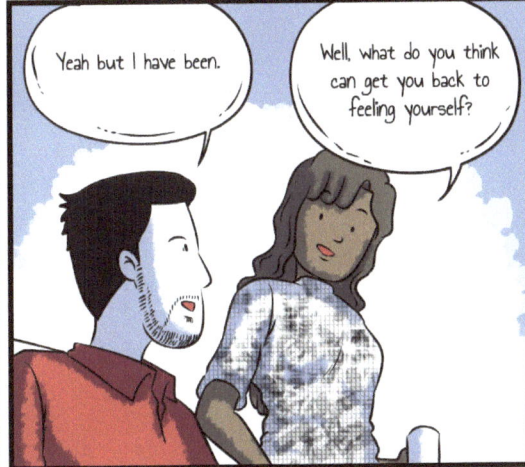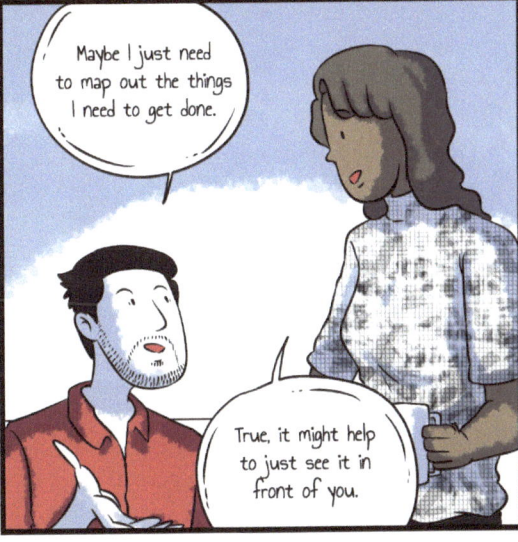

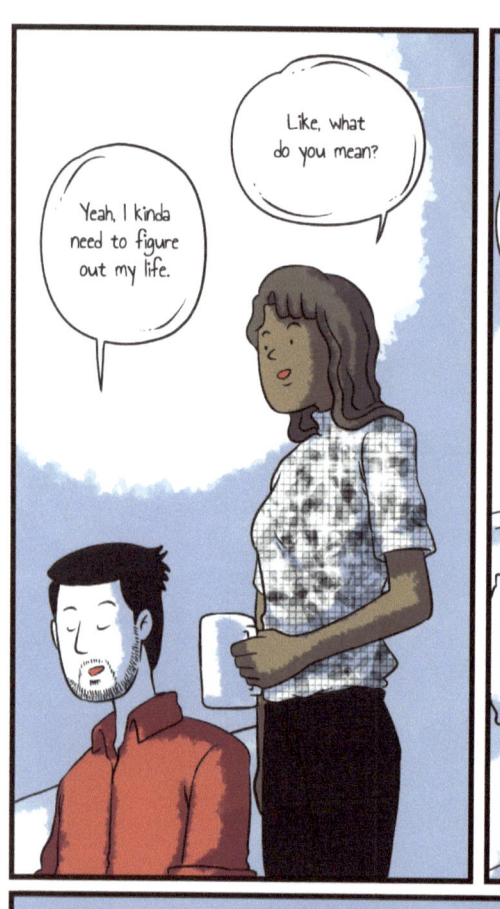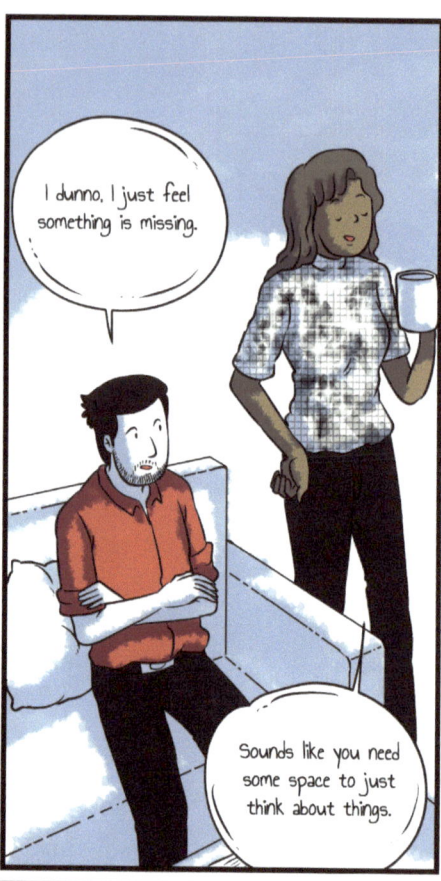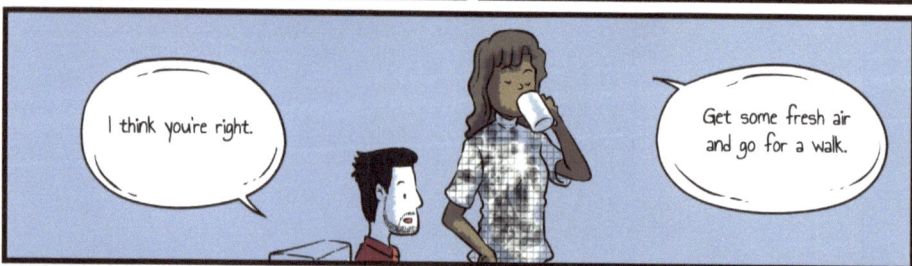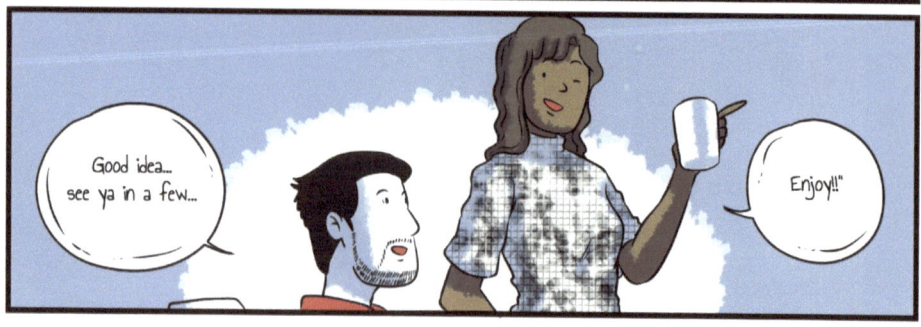

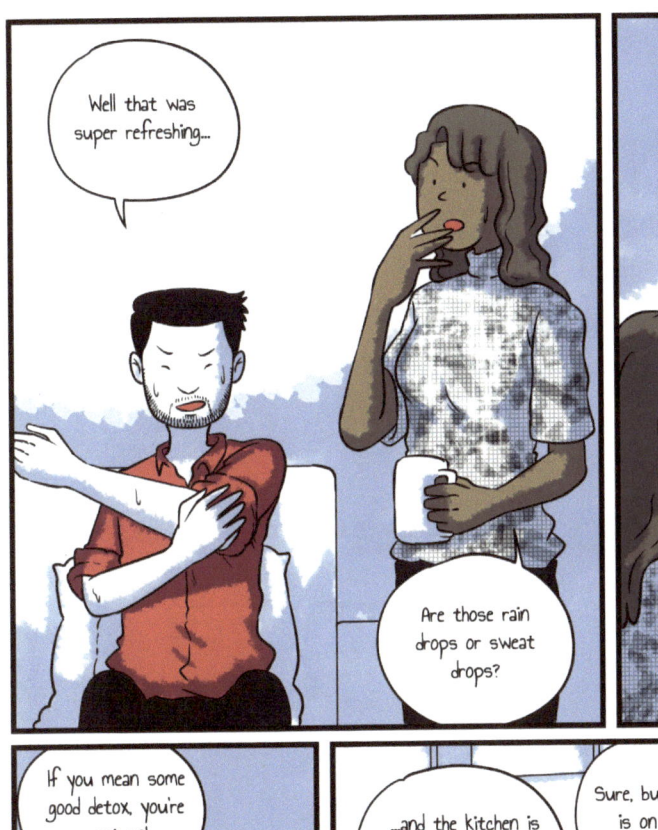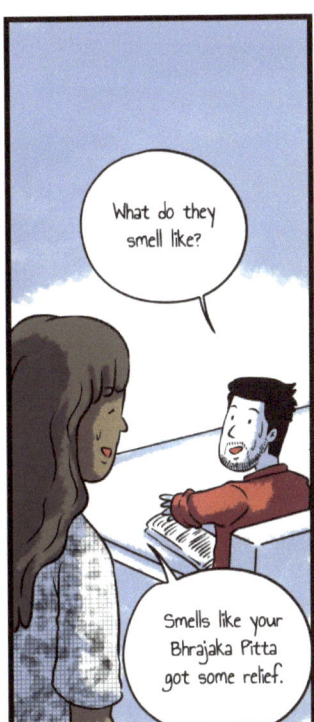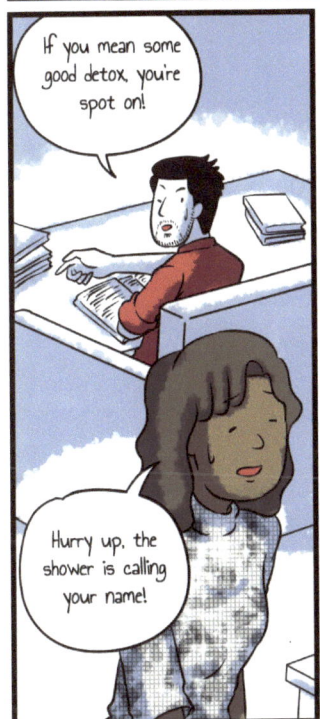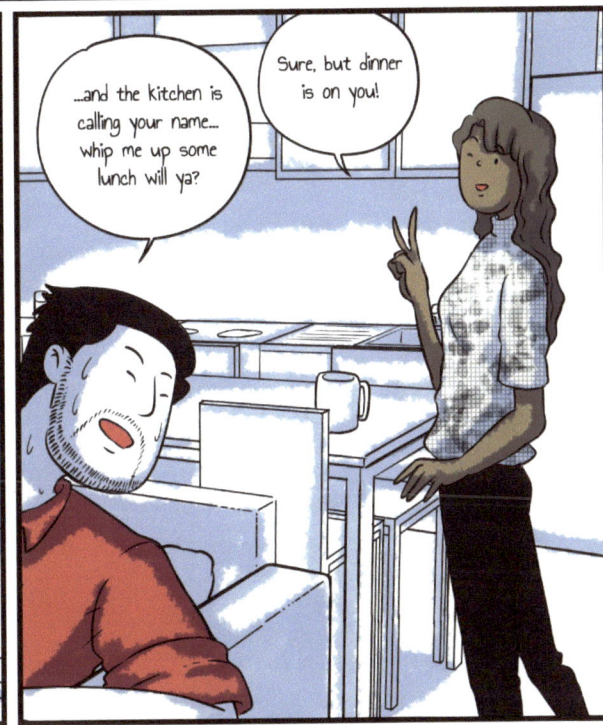

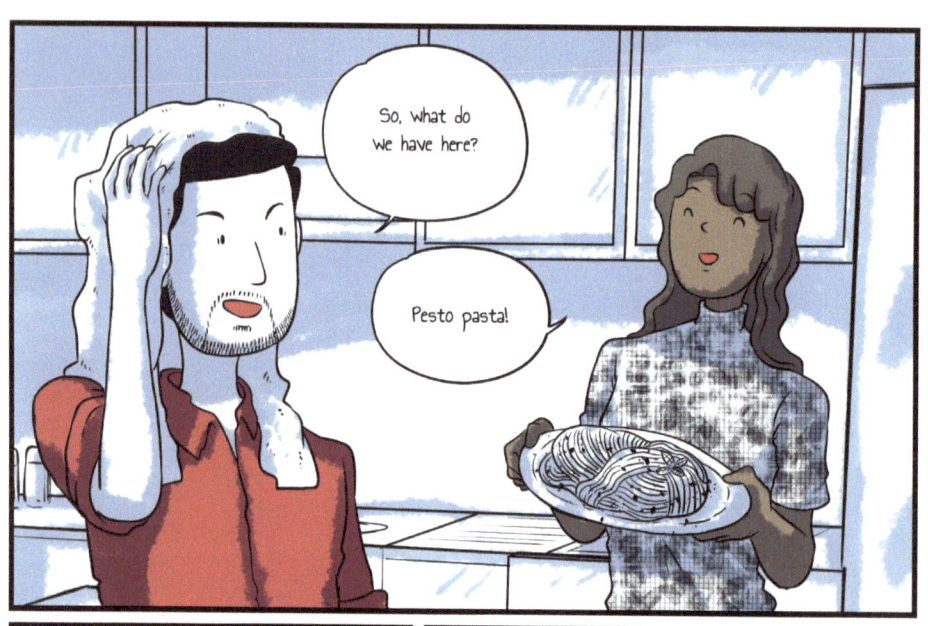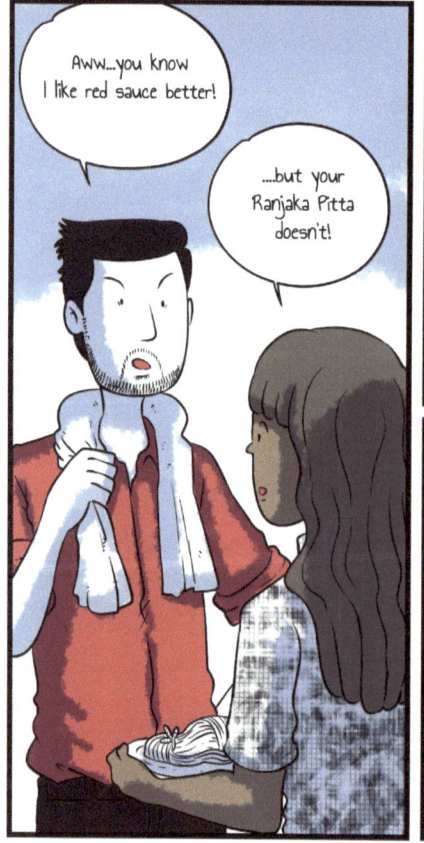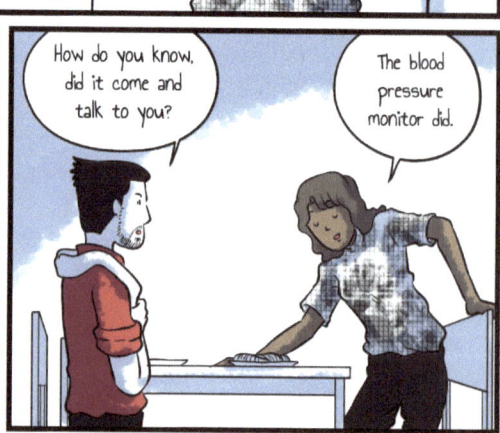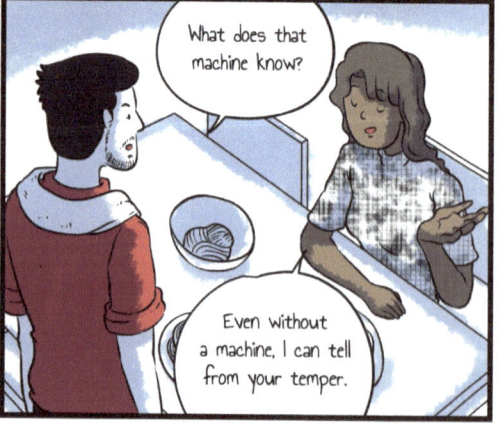

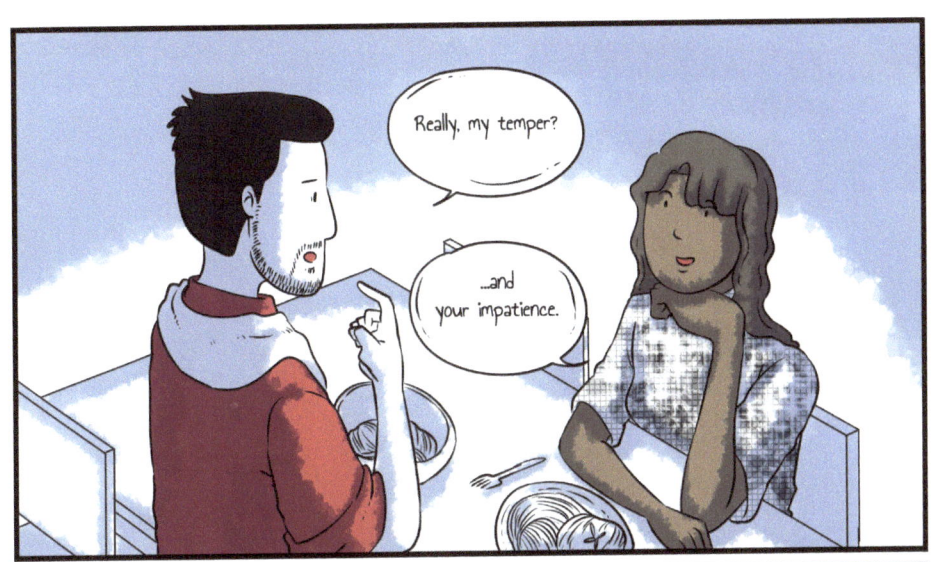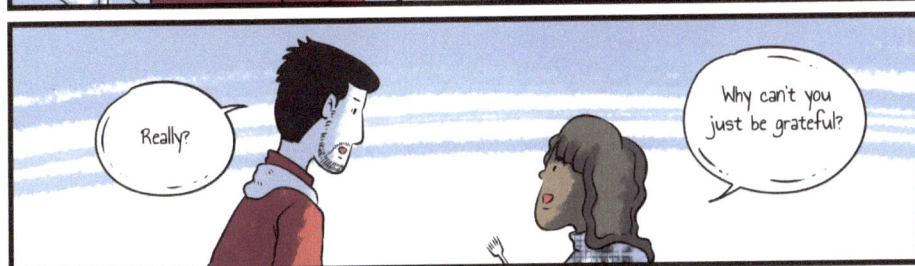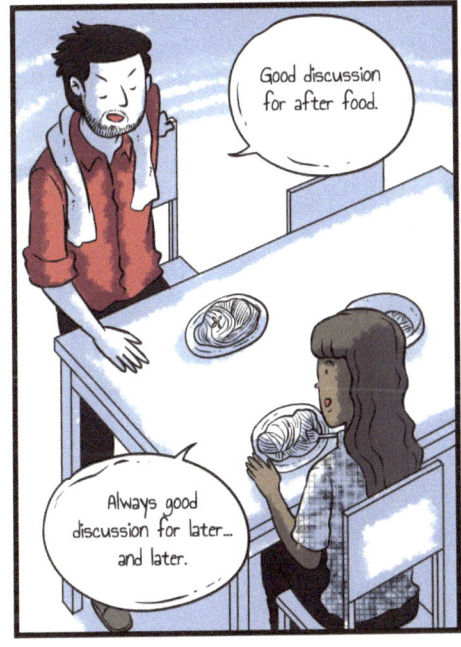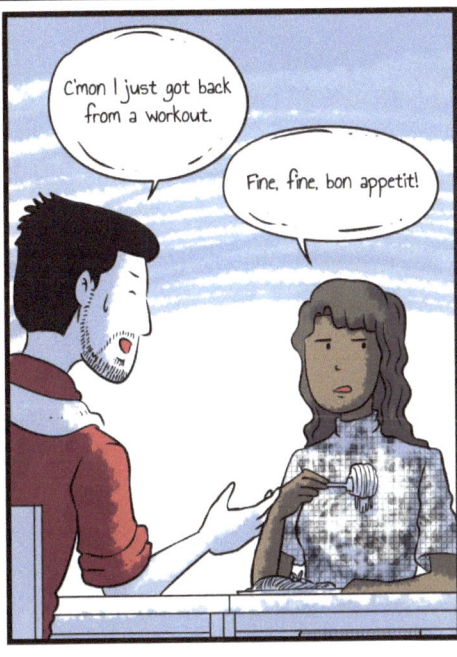

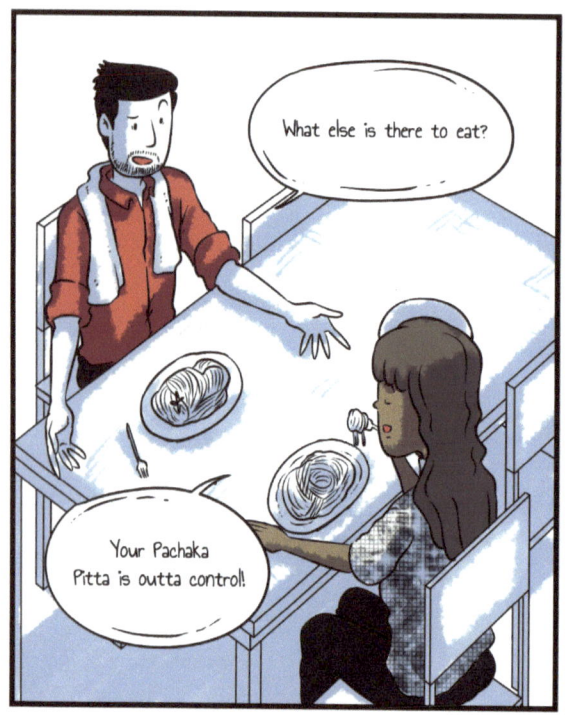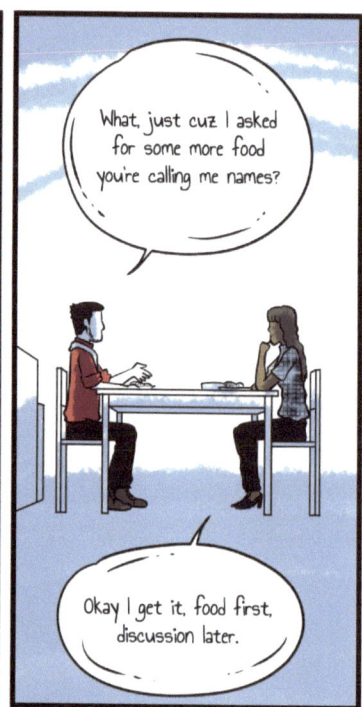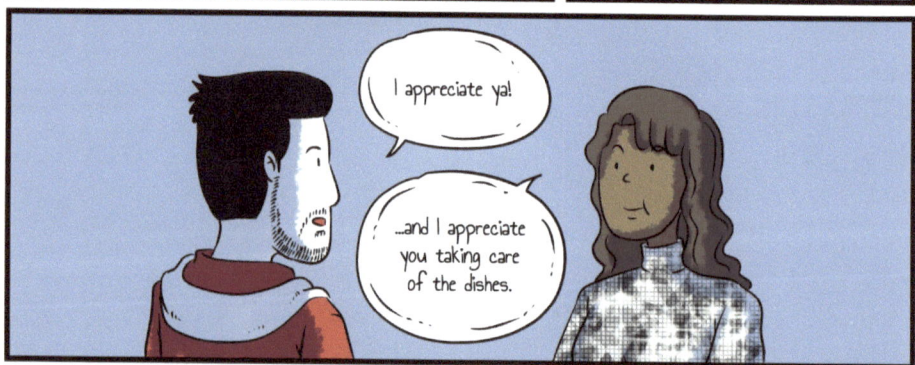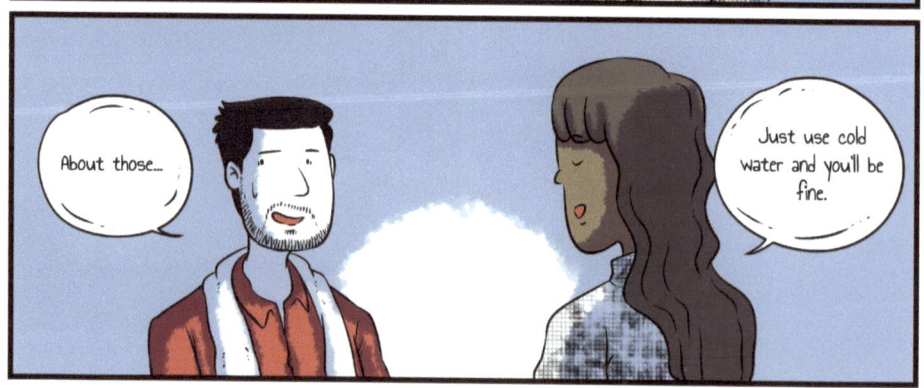

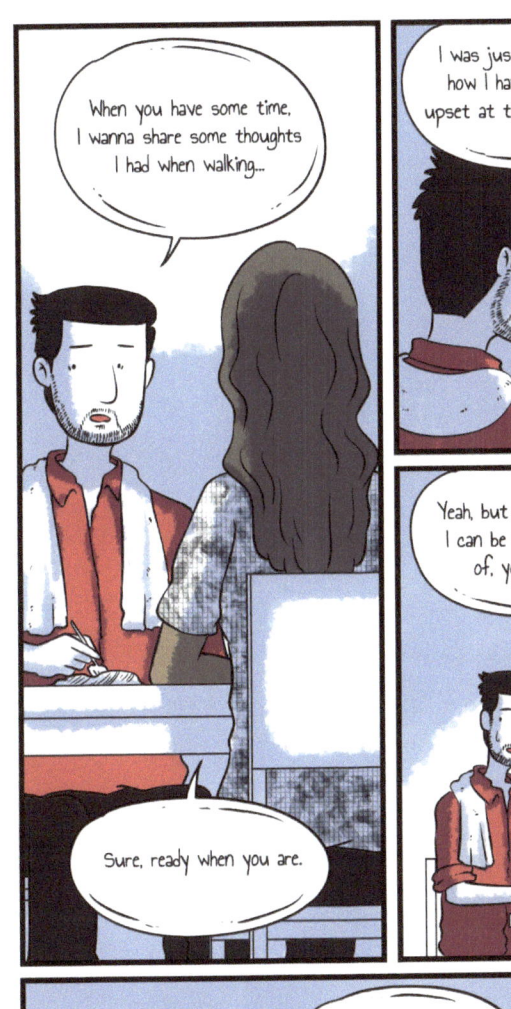
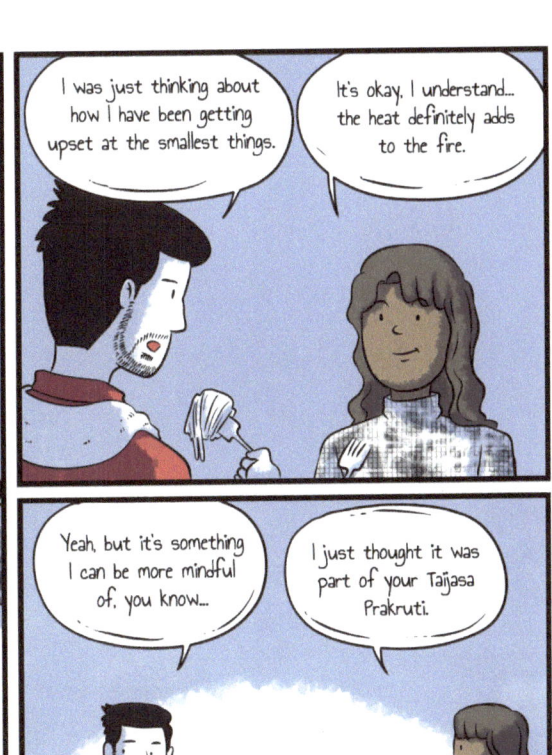
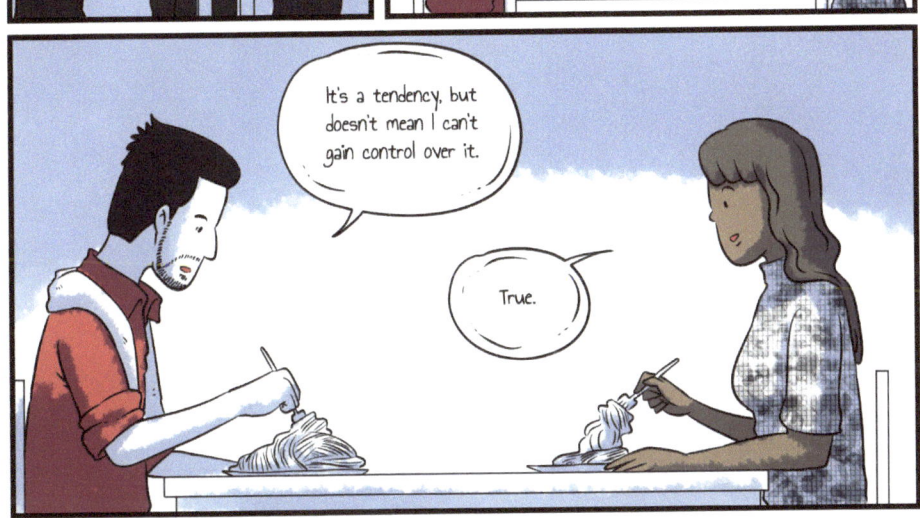

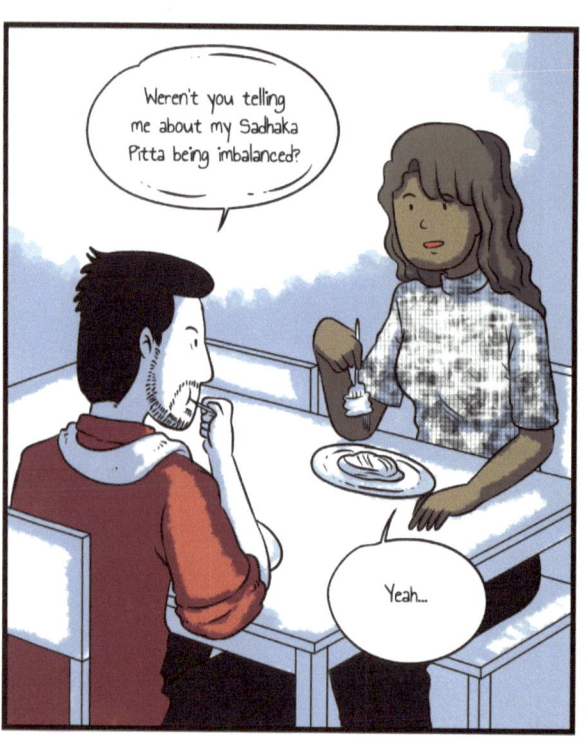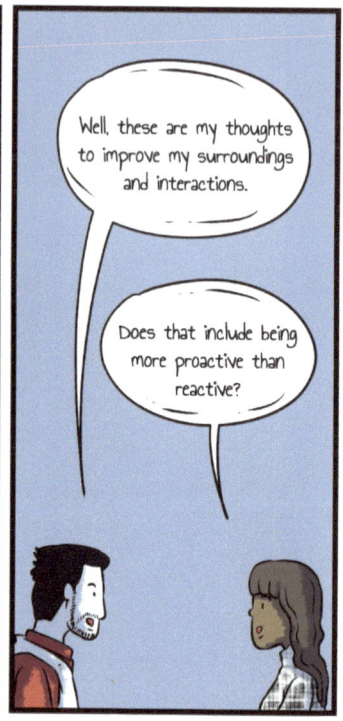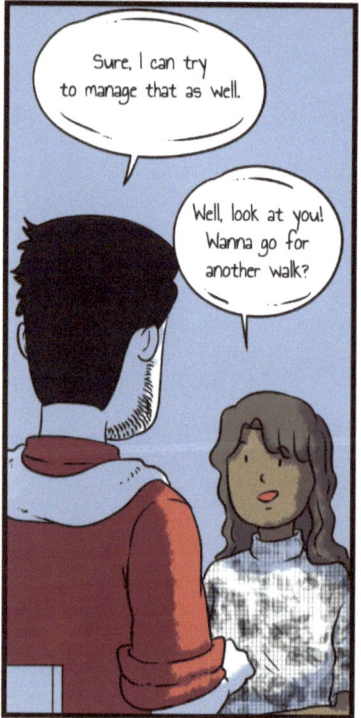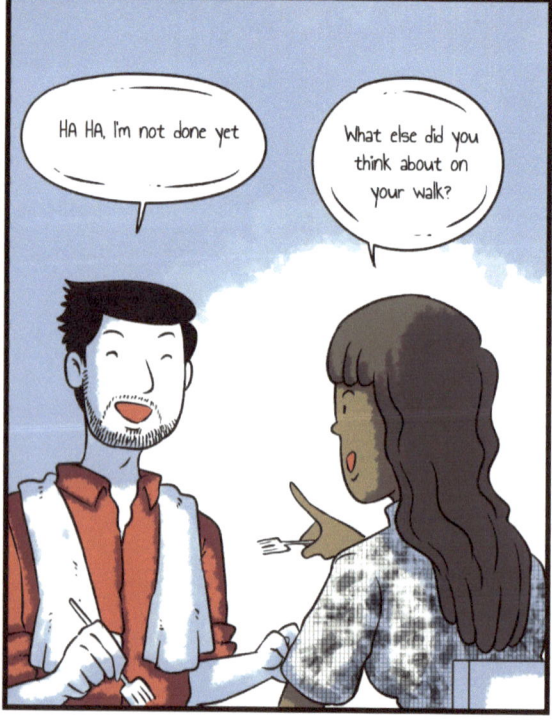

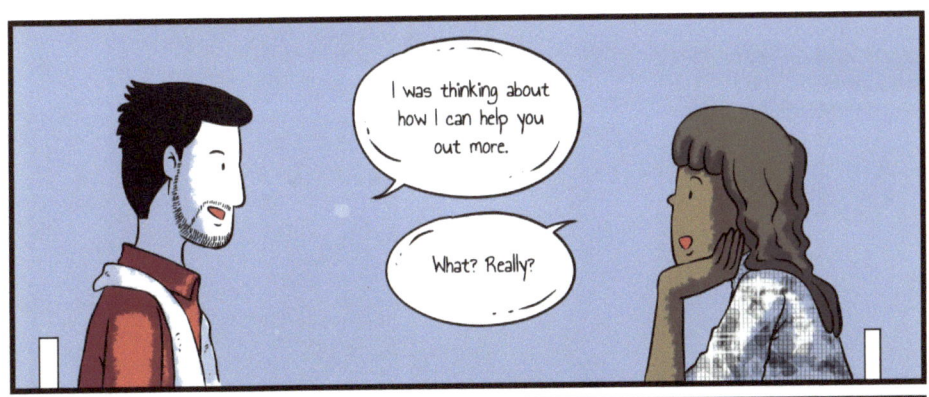
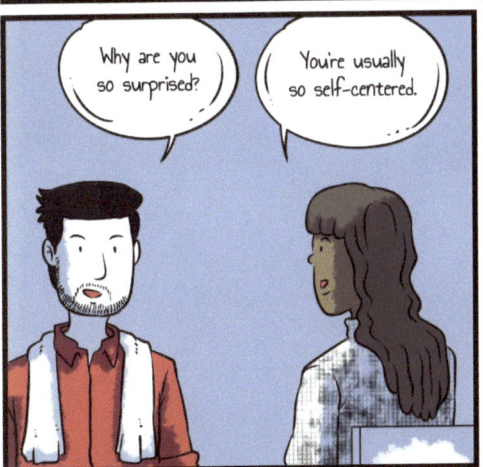
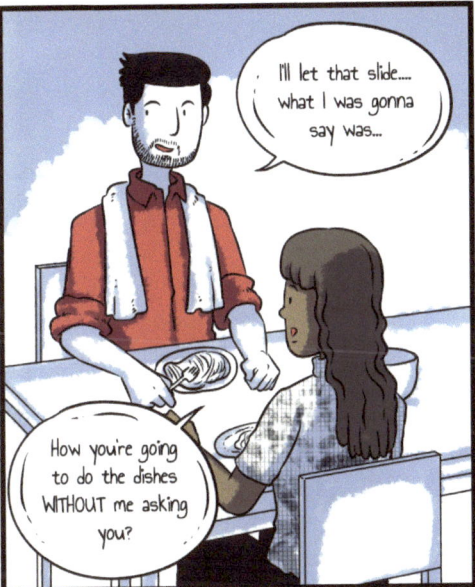
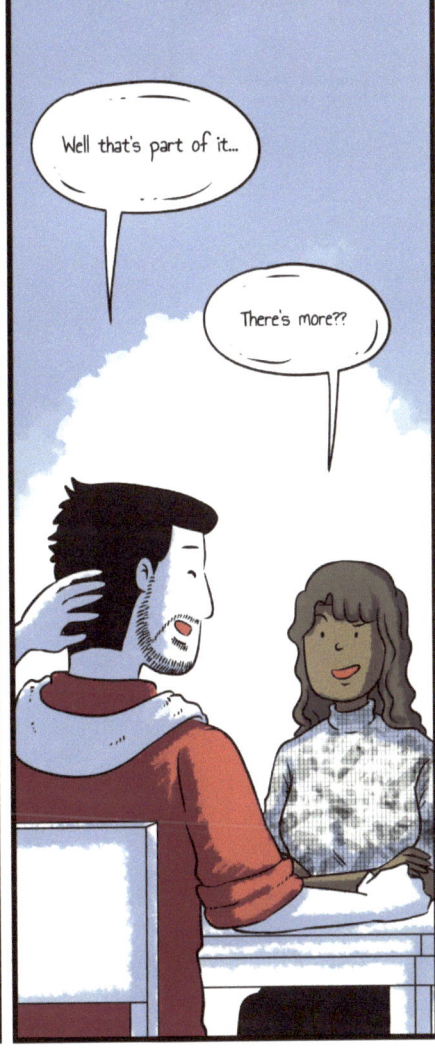

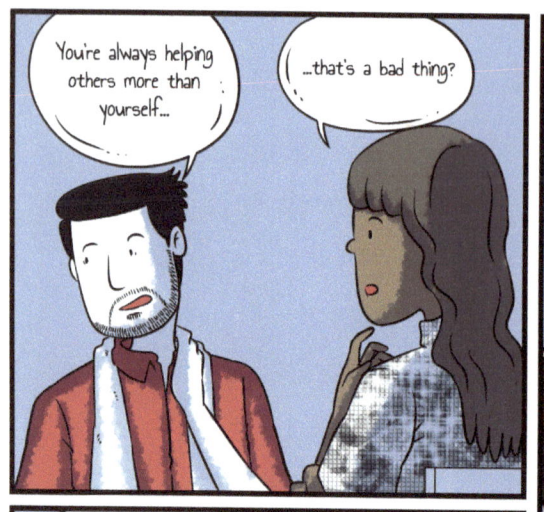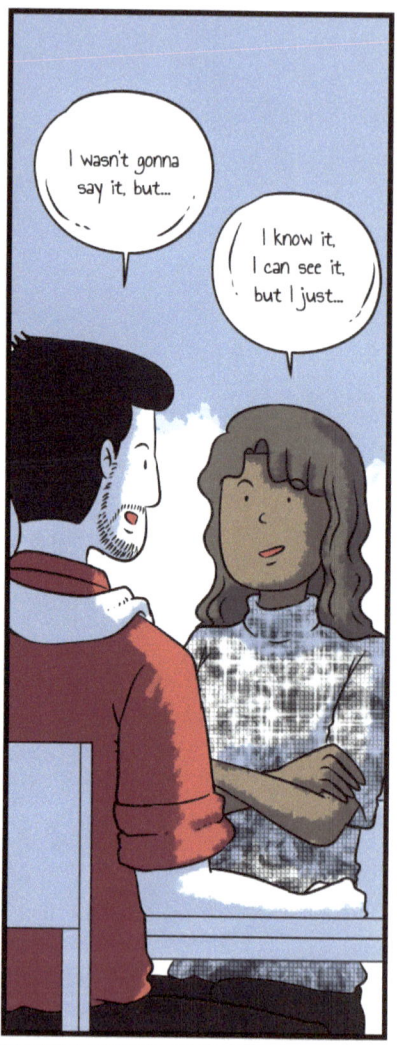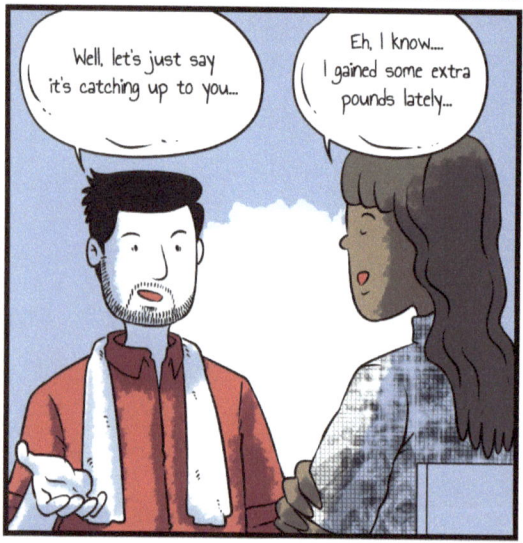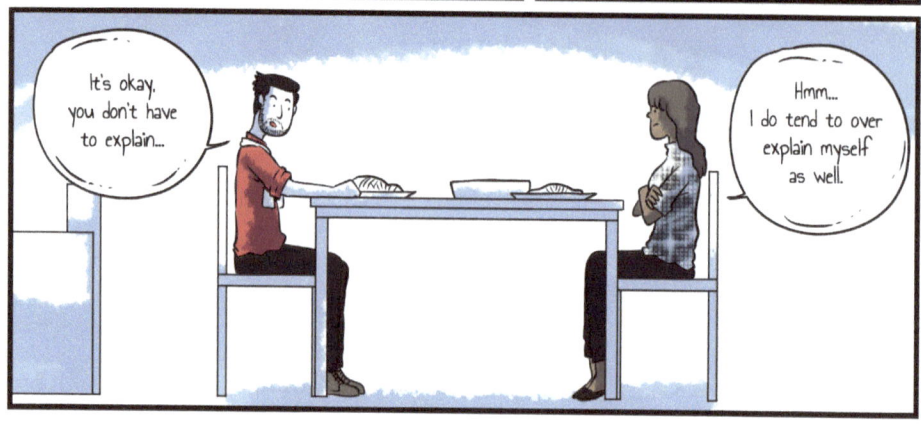

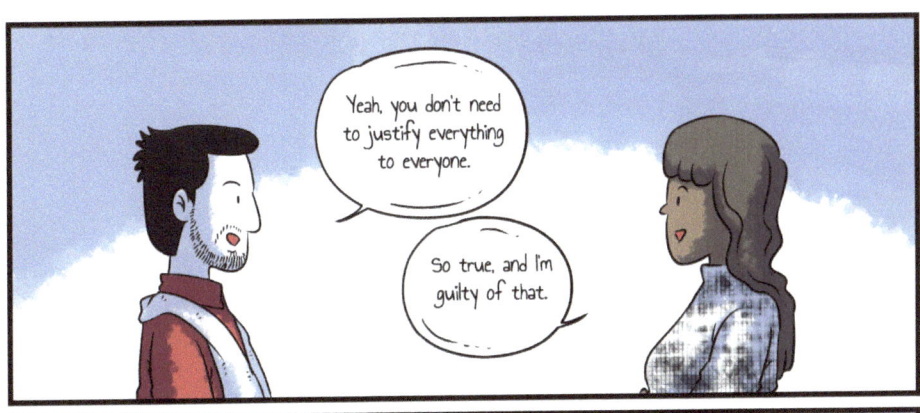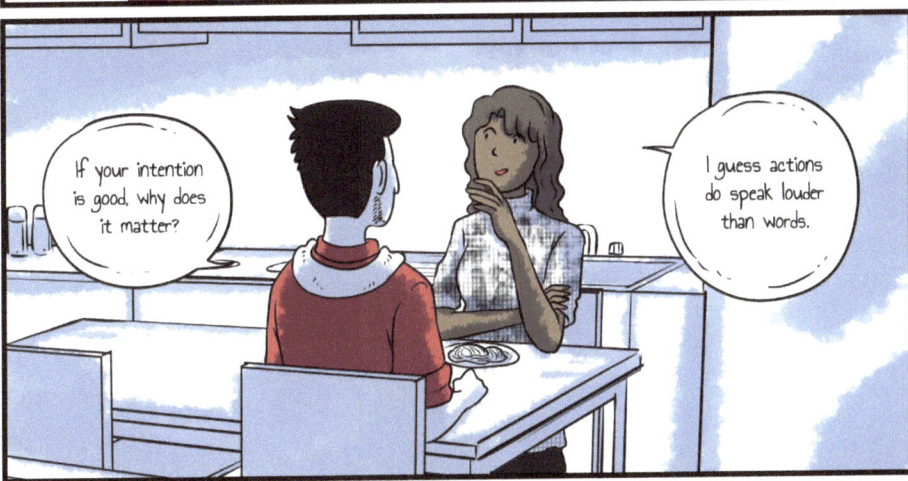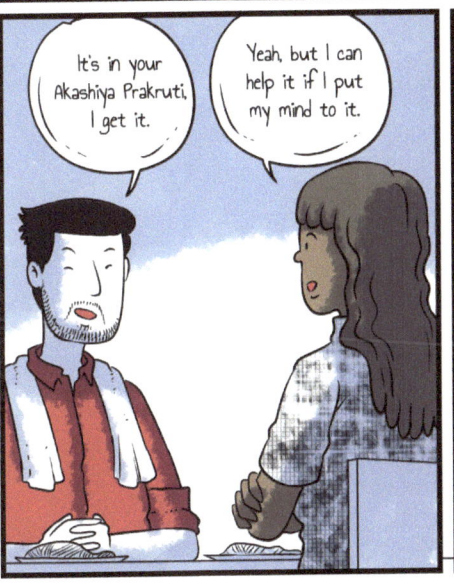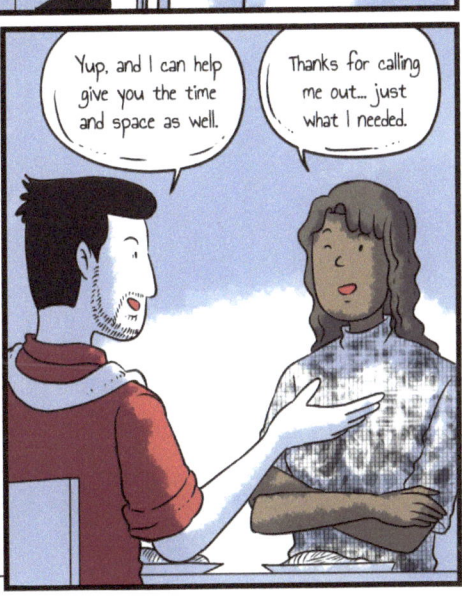

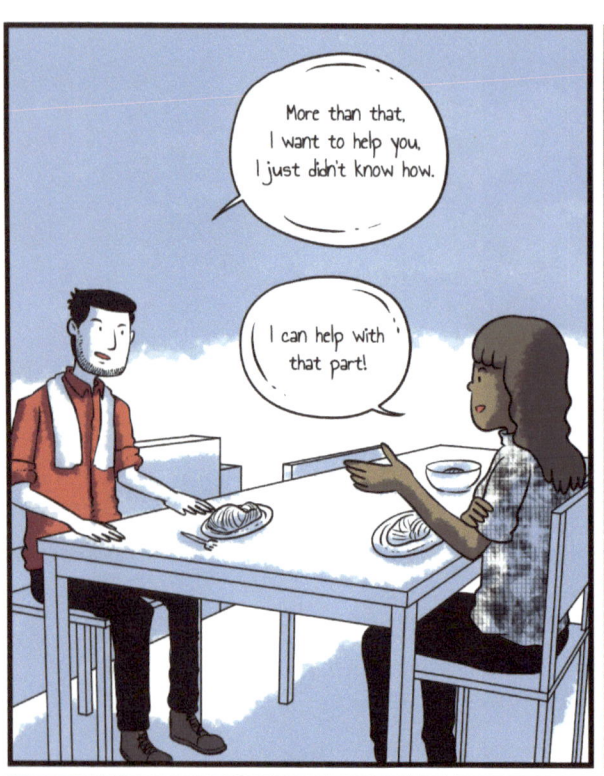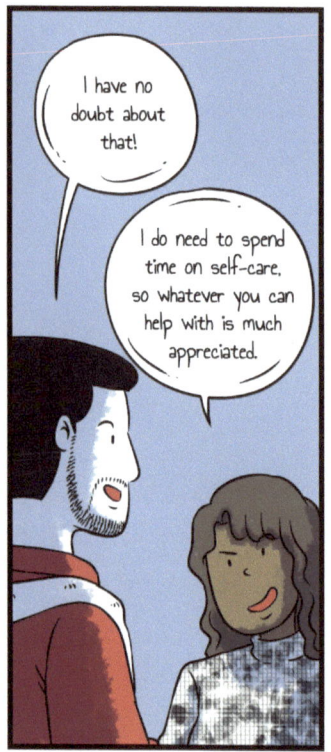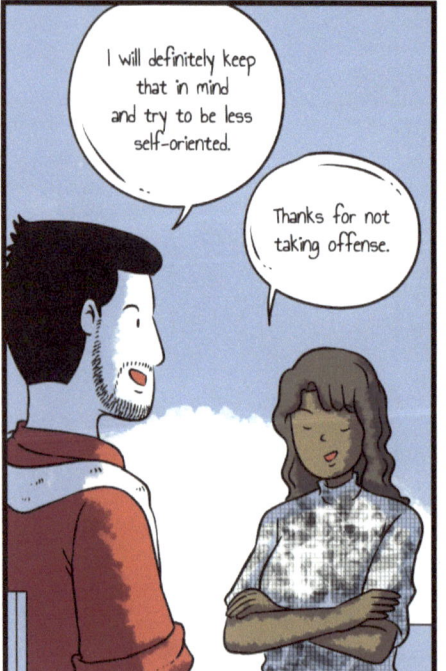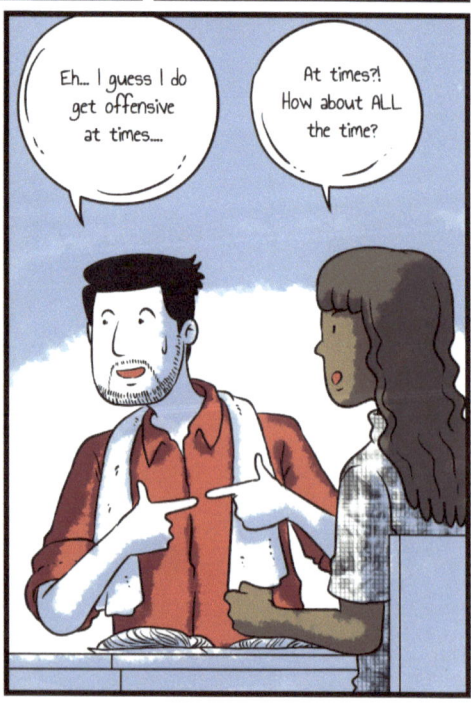

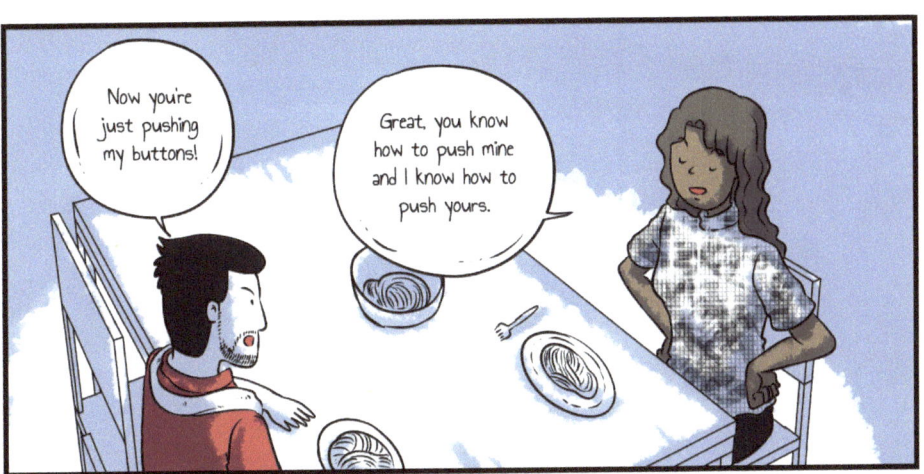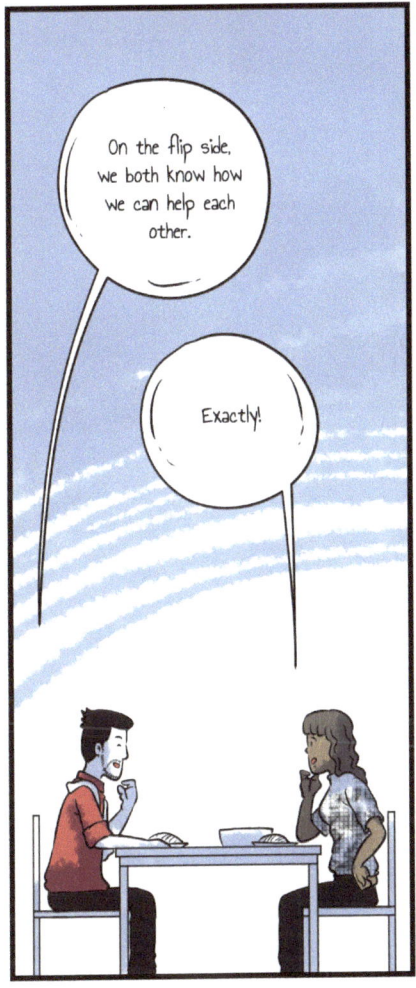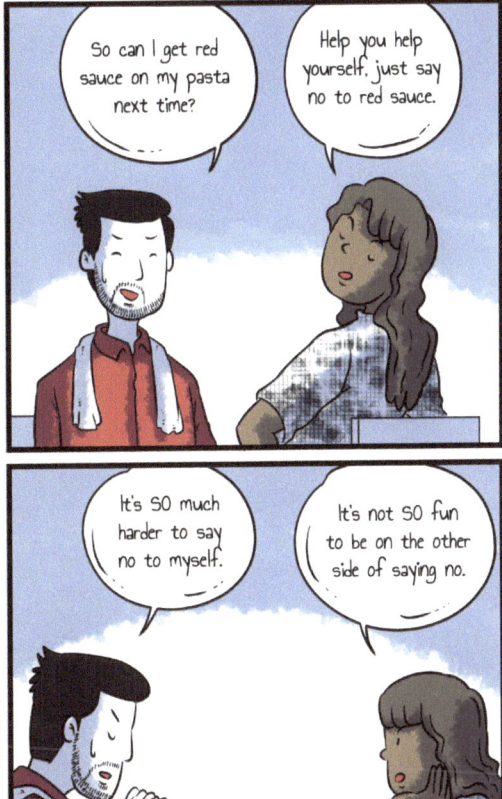

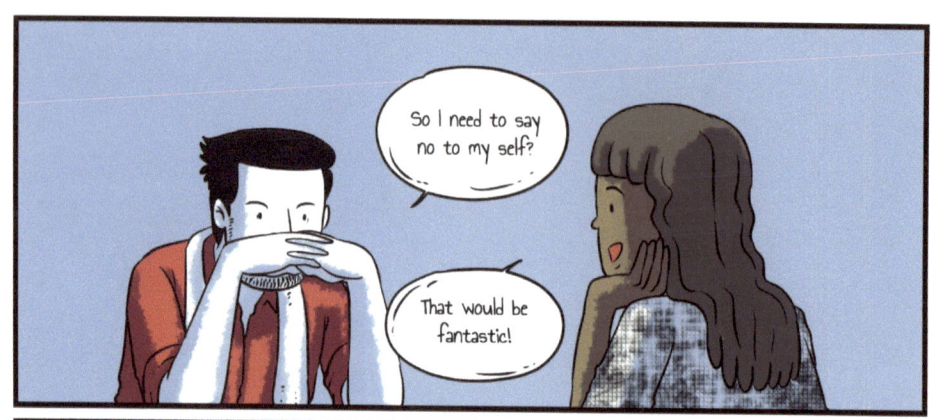
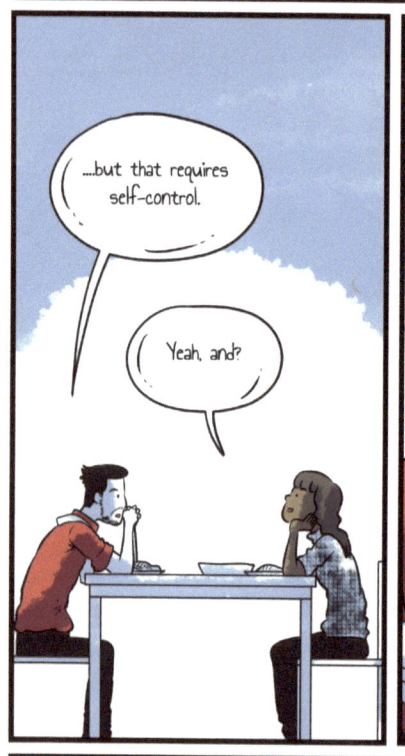
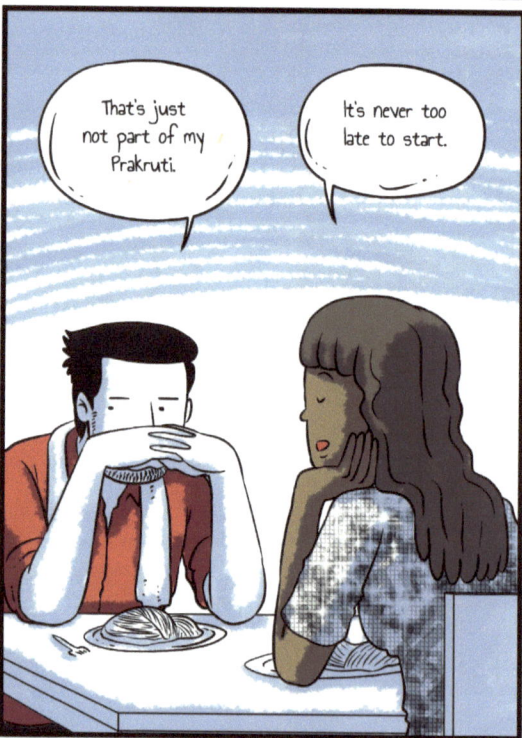
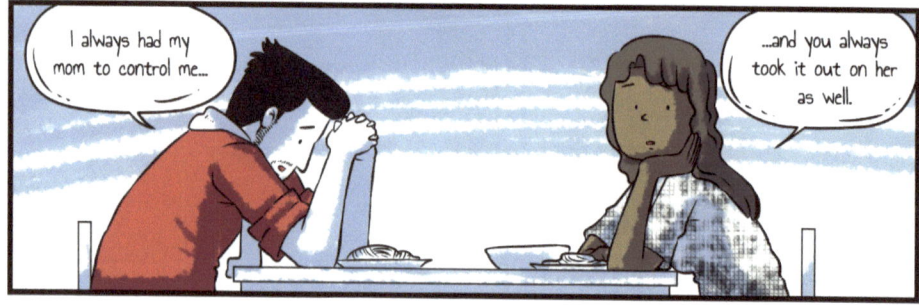

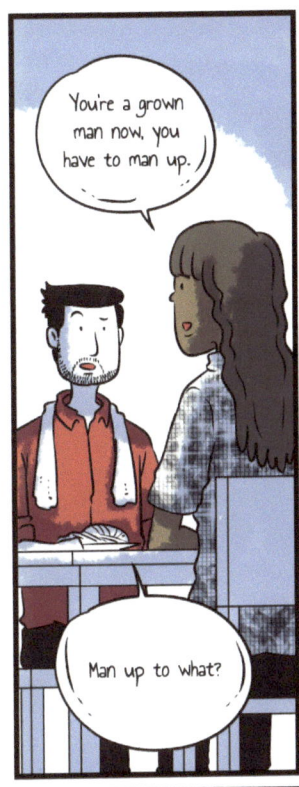
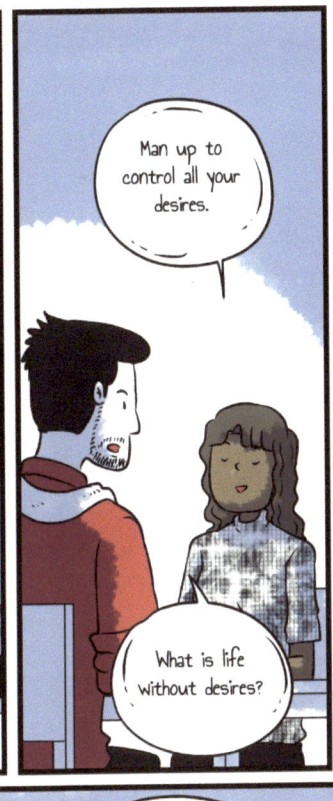
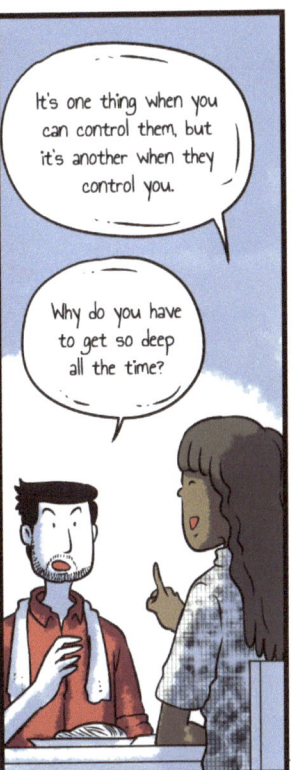
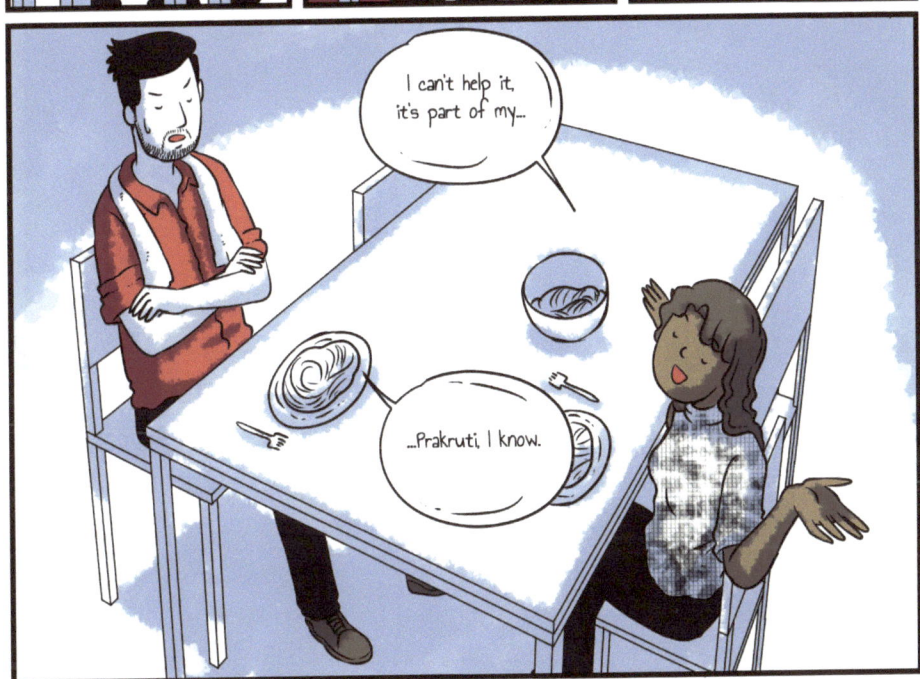

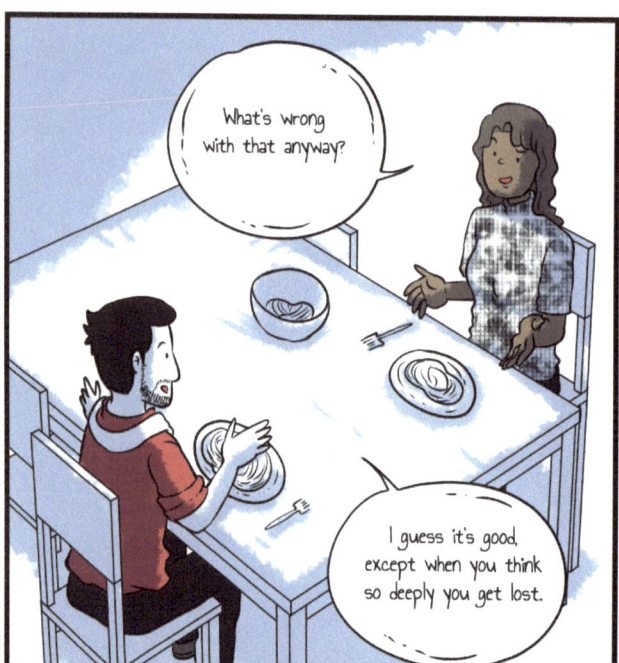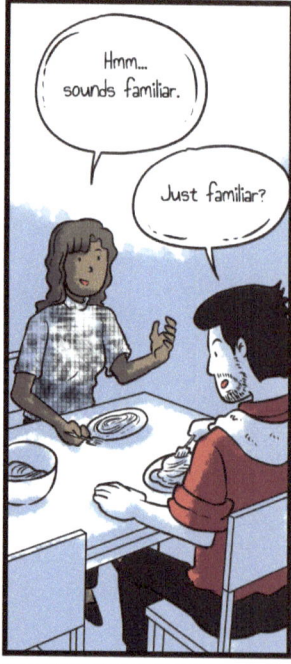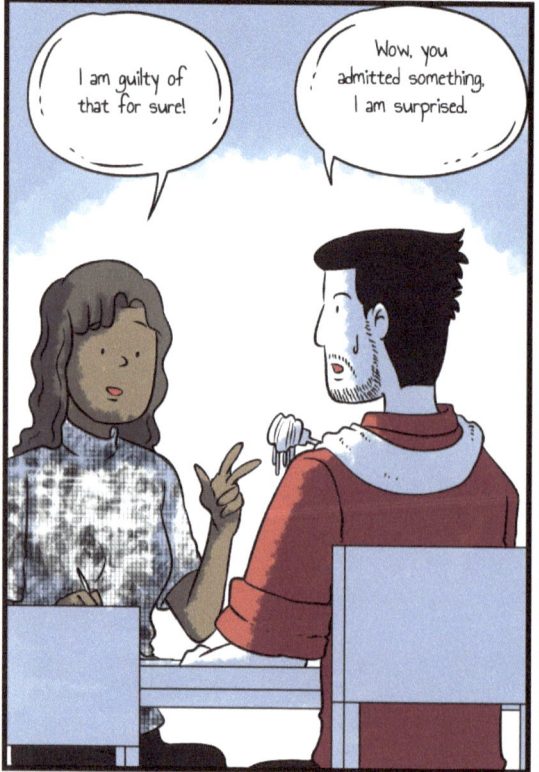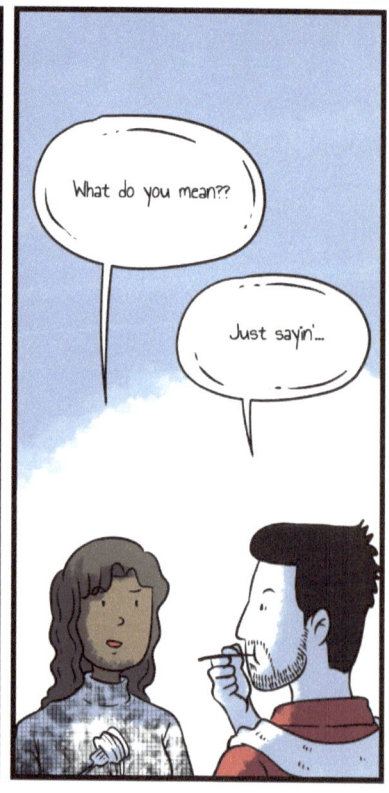

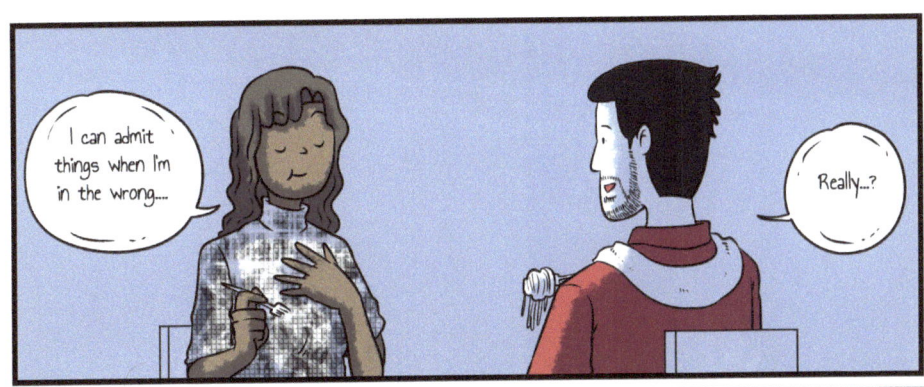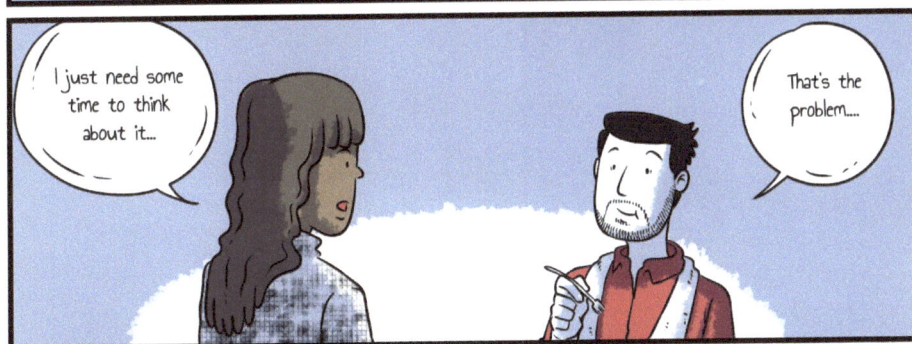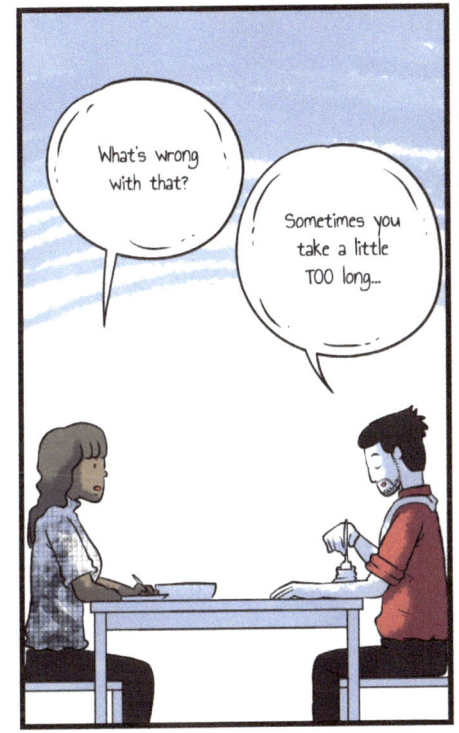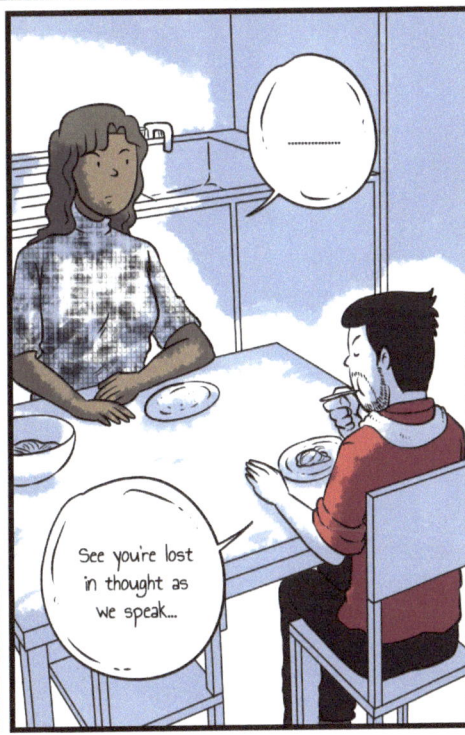

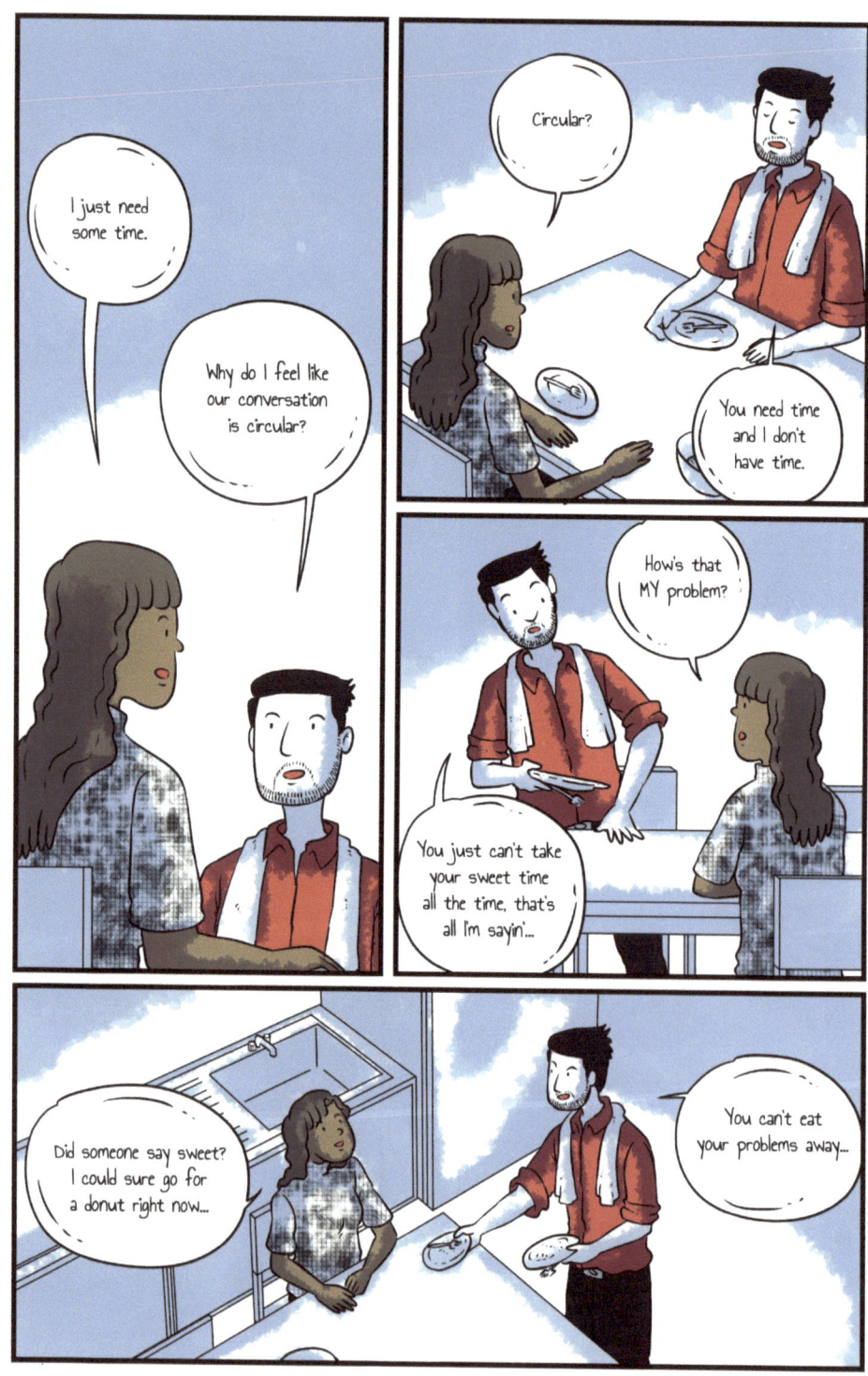

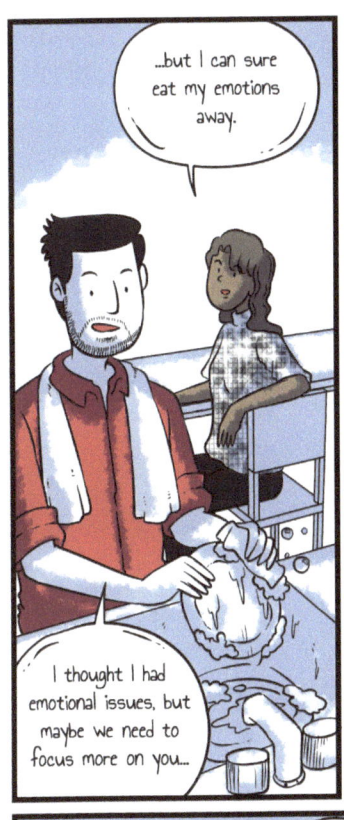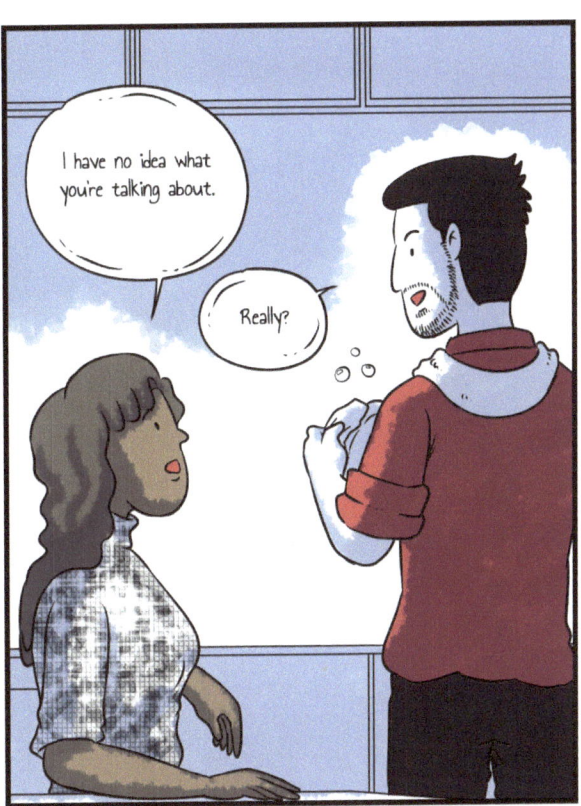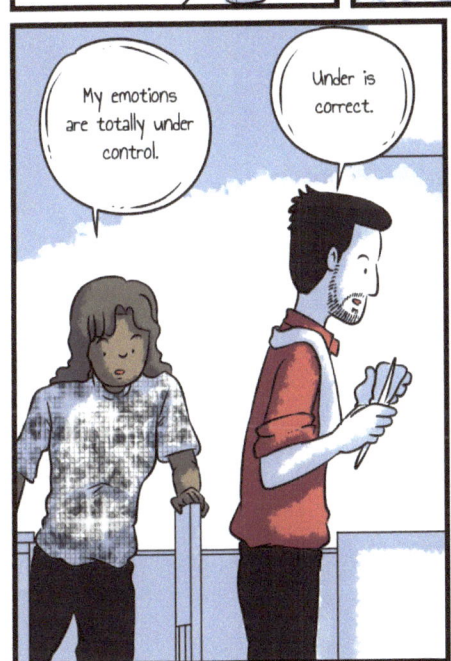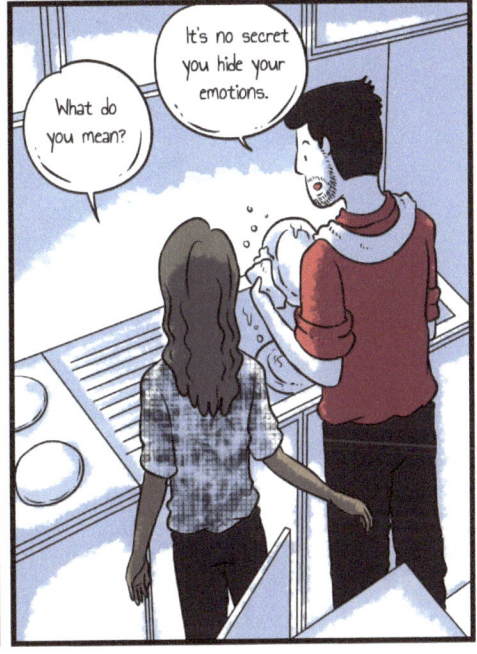

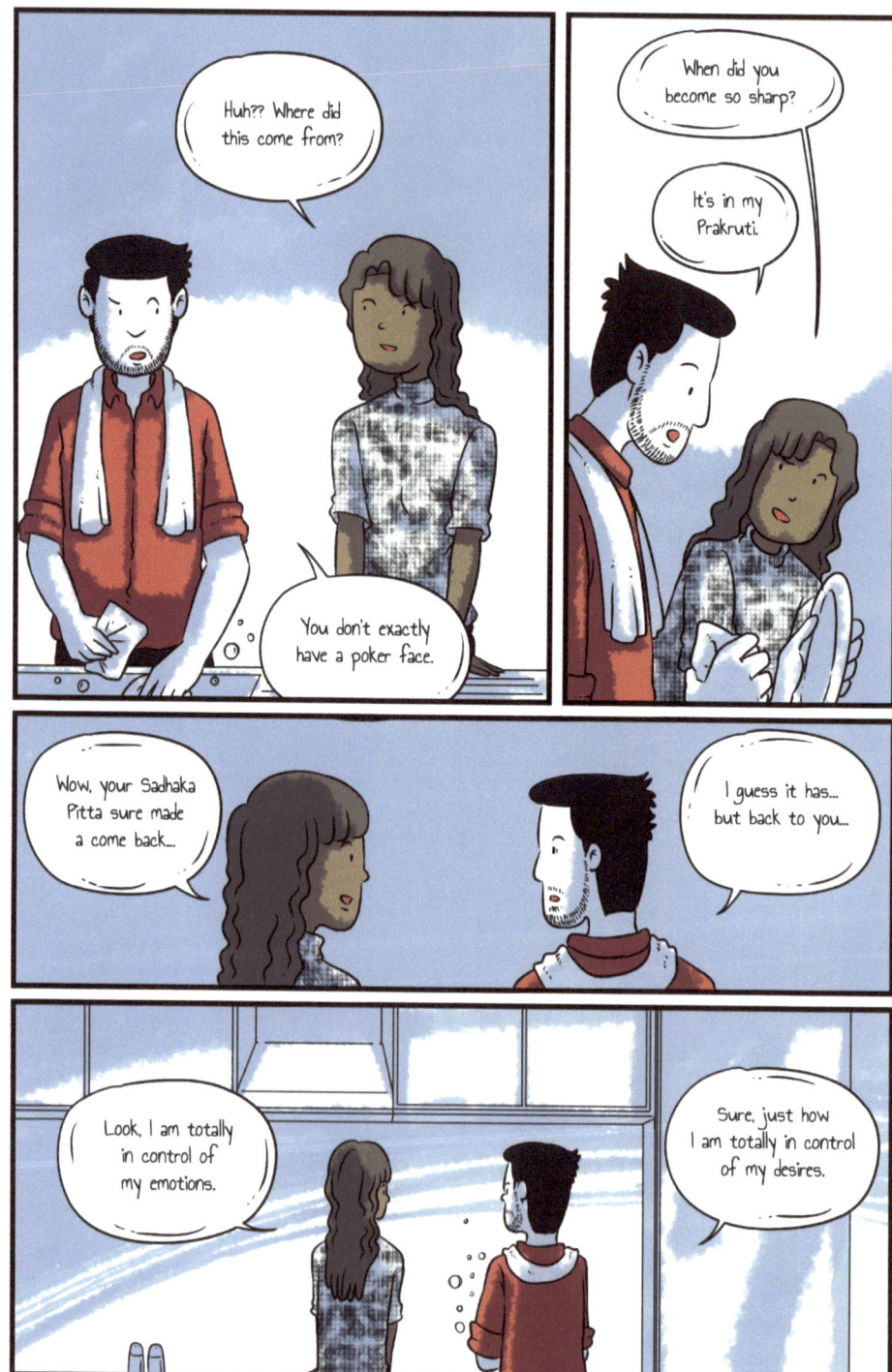

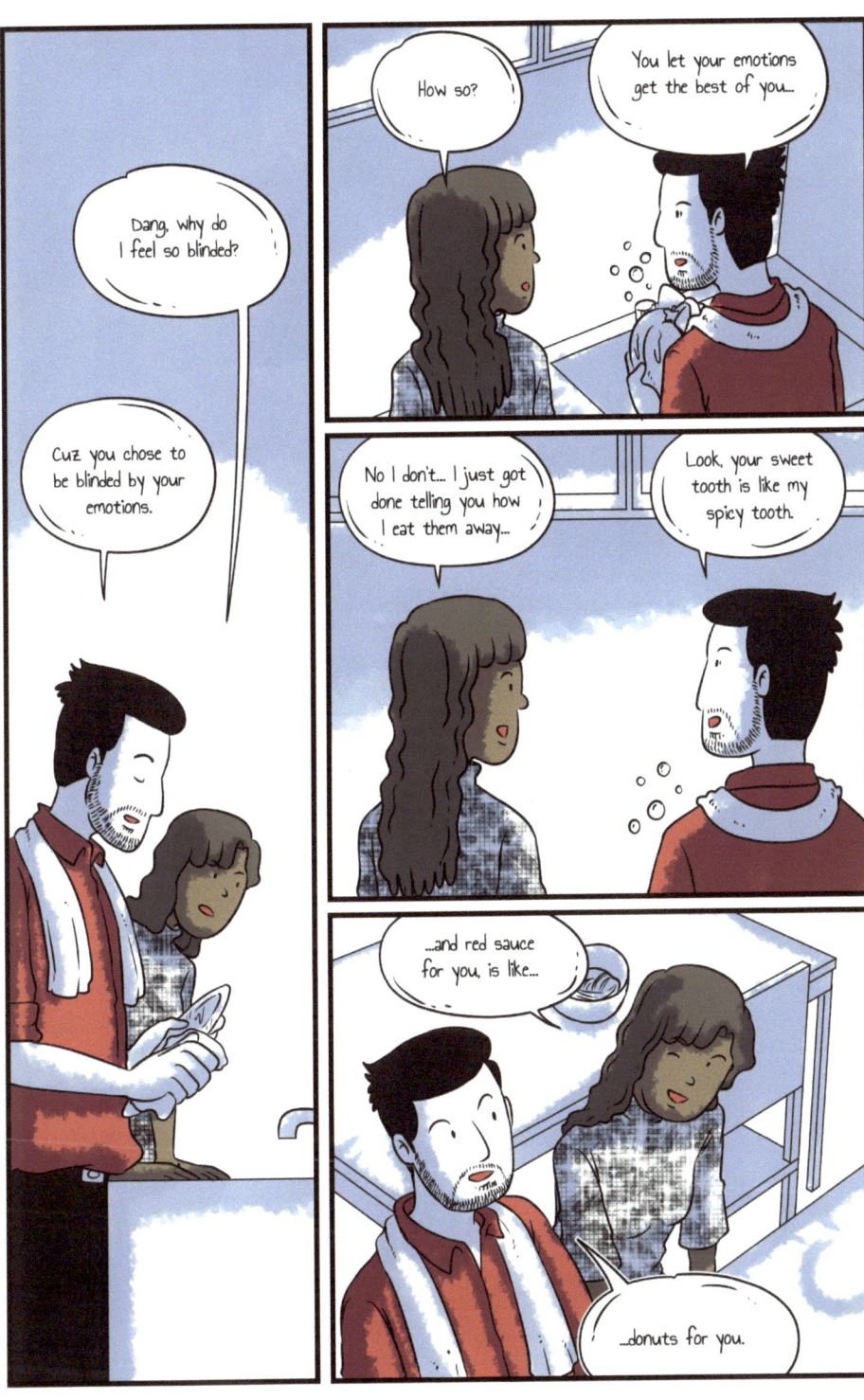

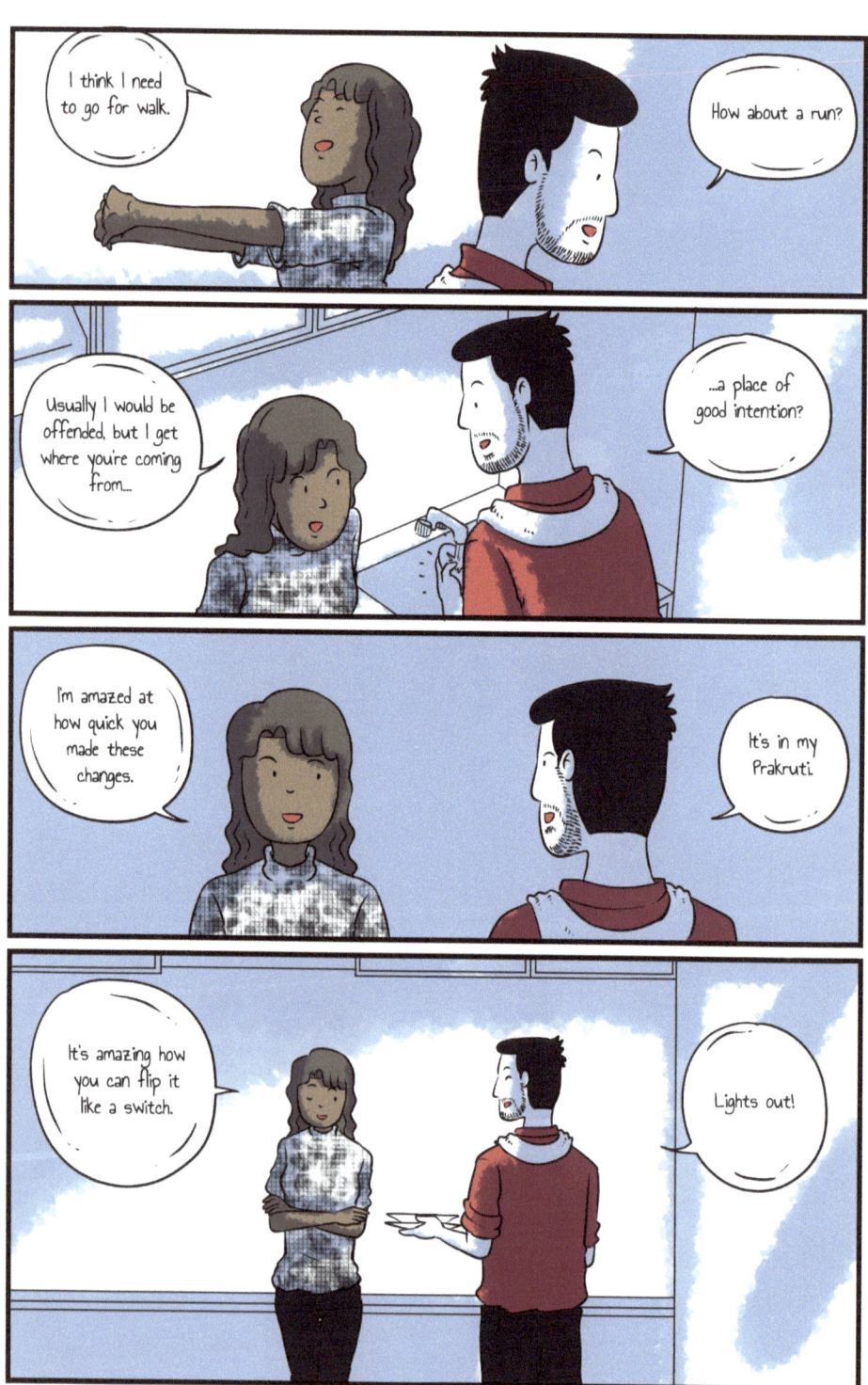

Section 3: Kapha

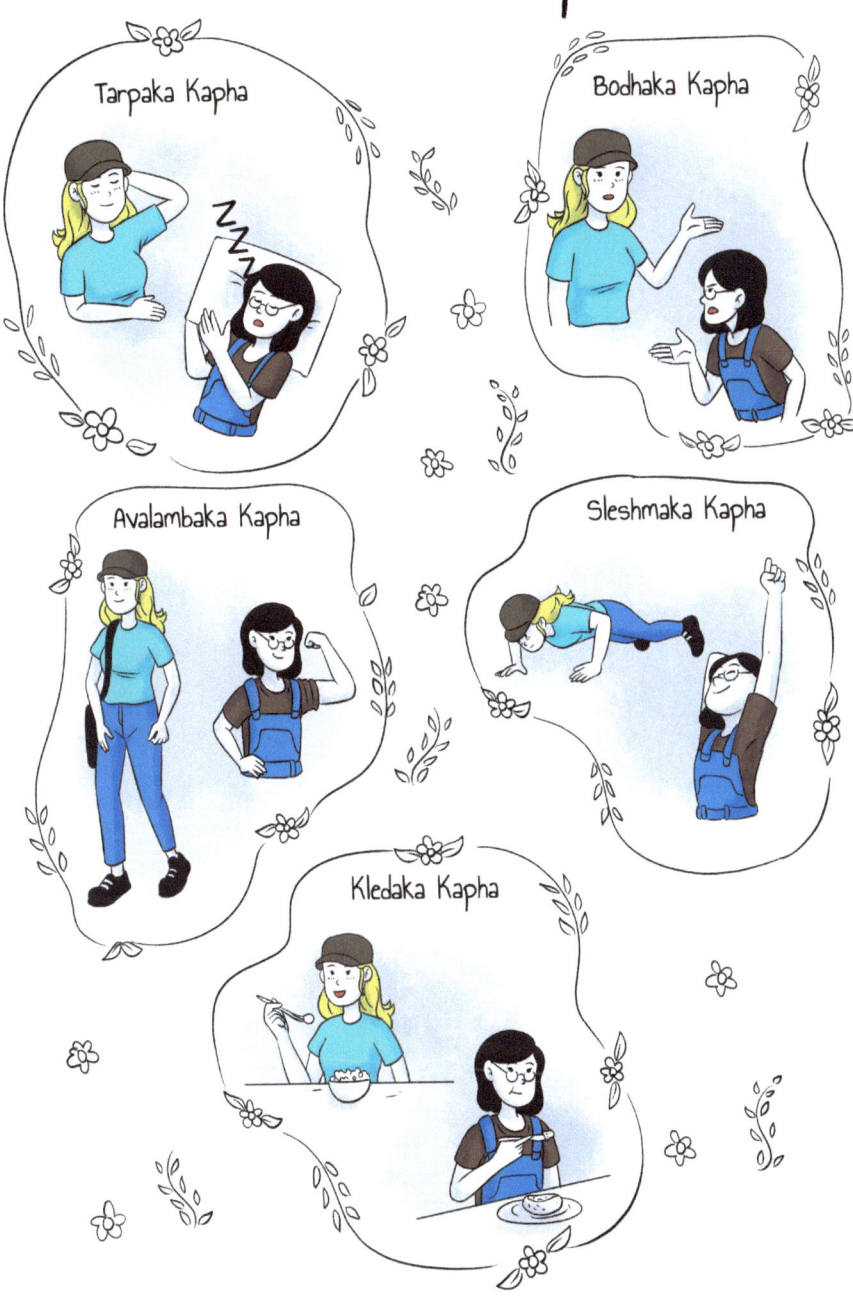

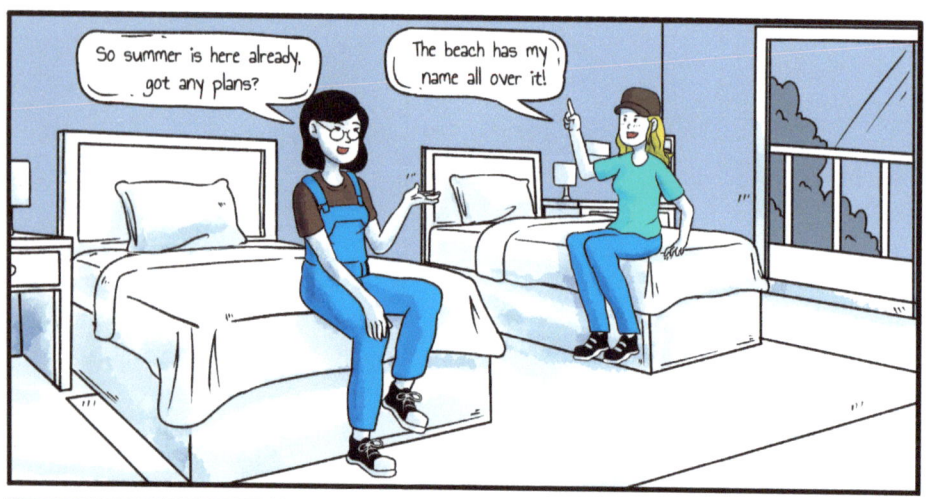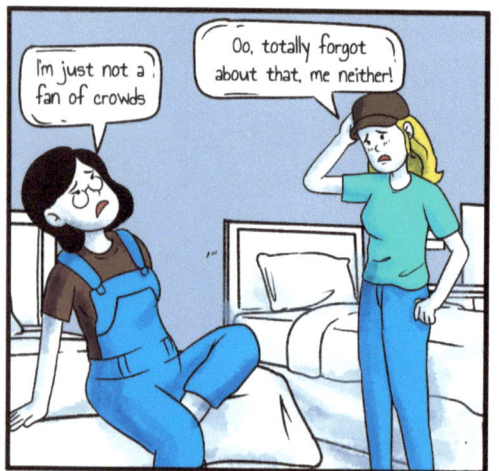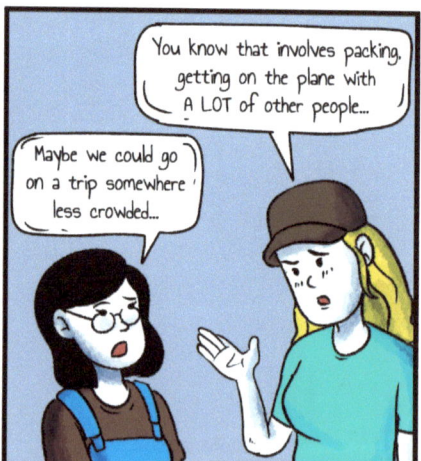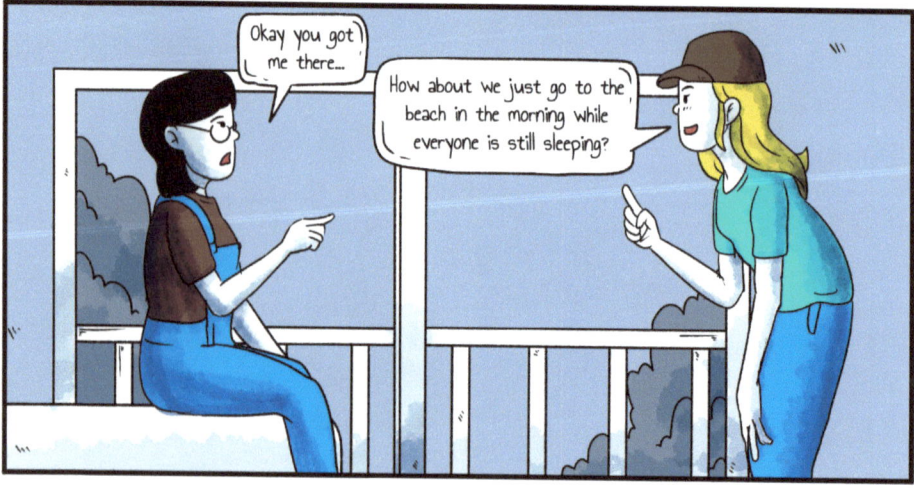

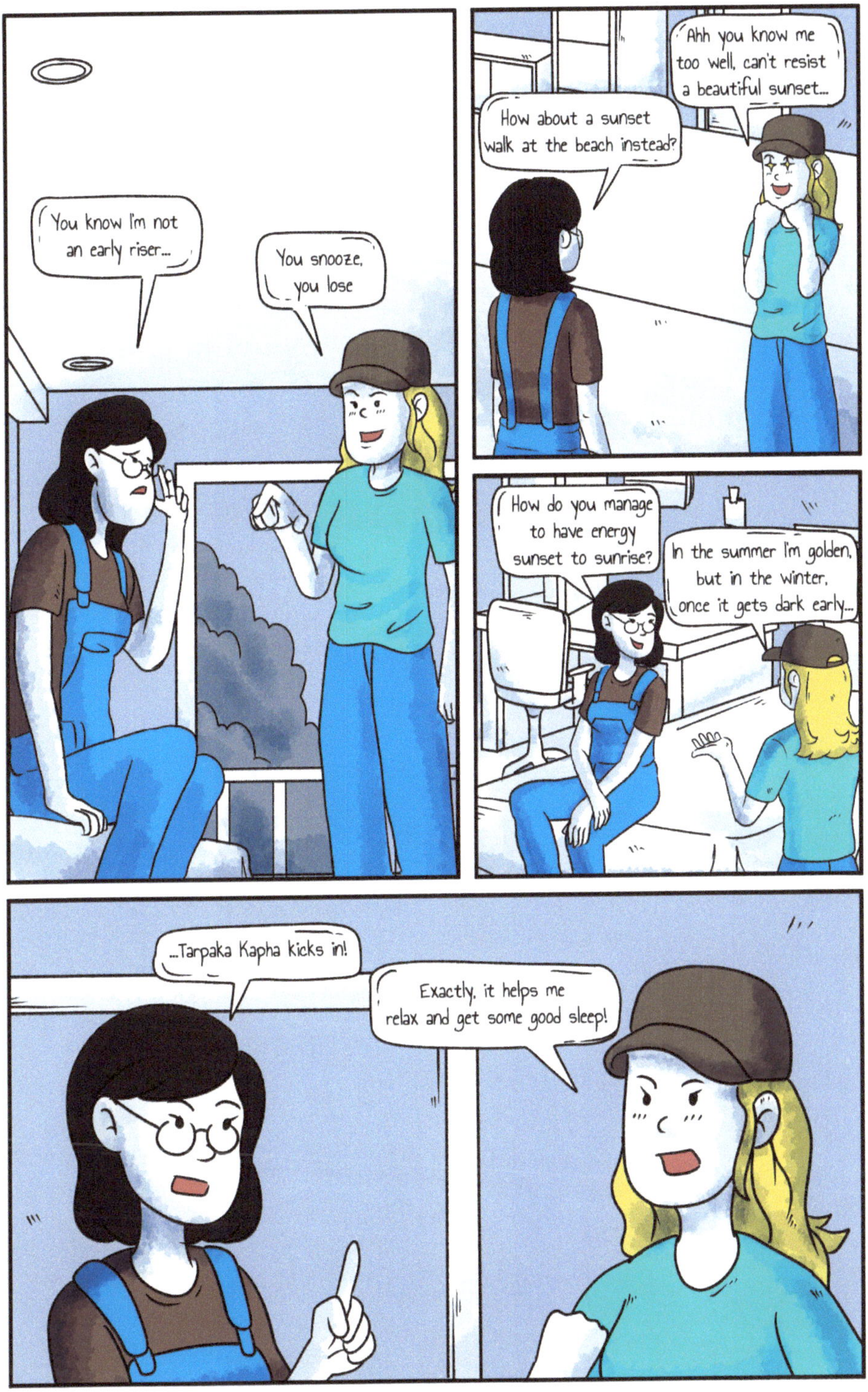

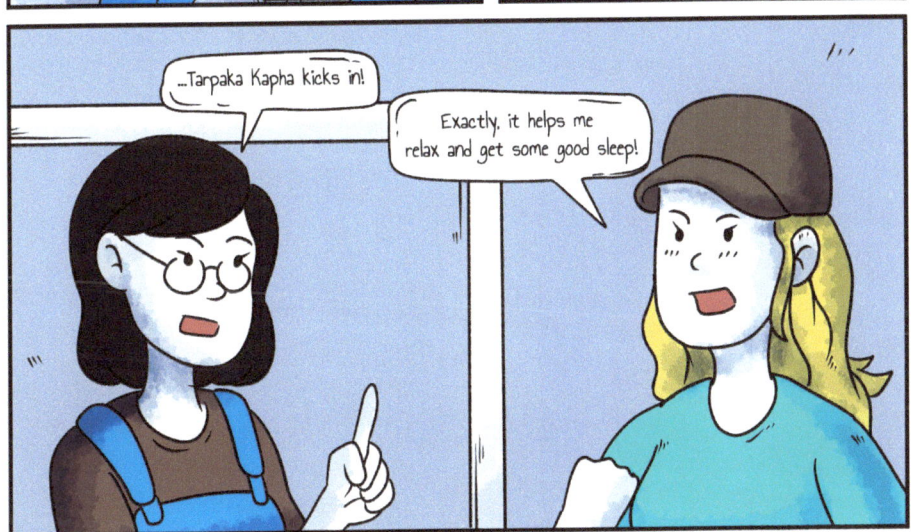

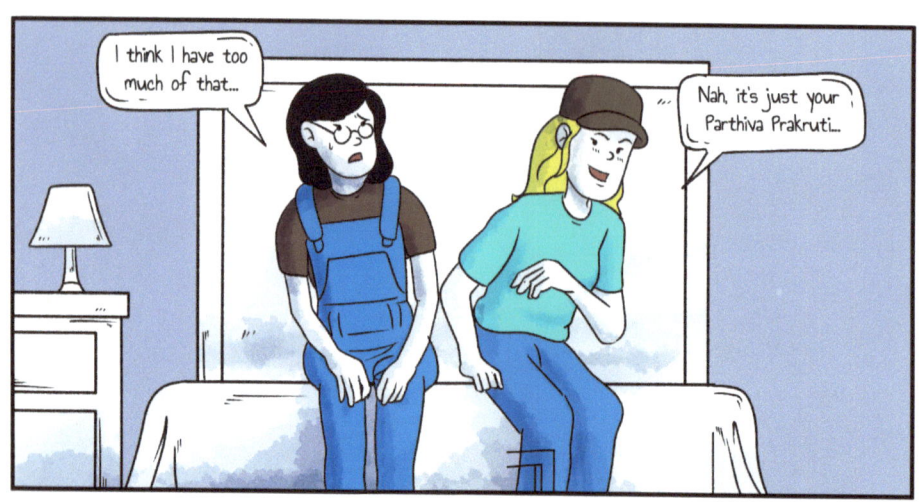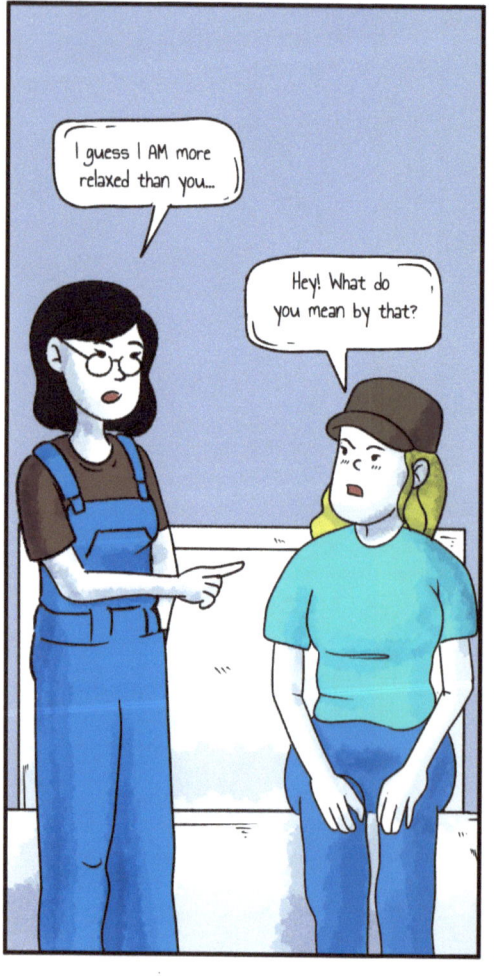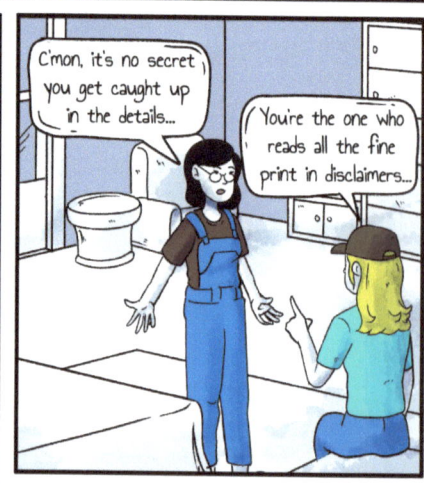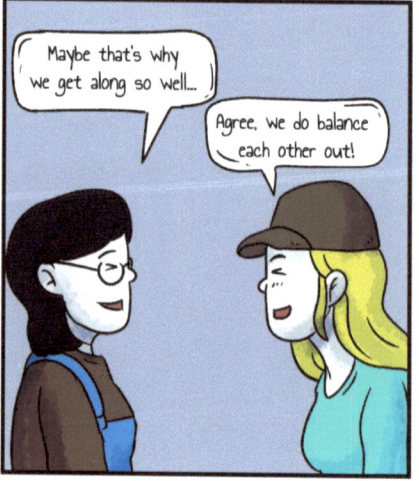

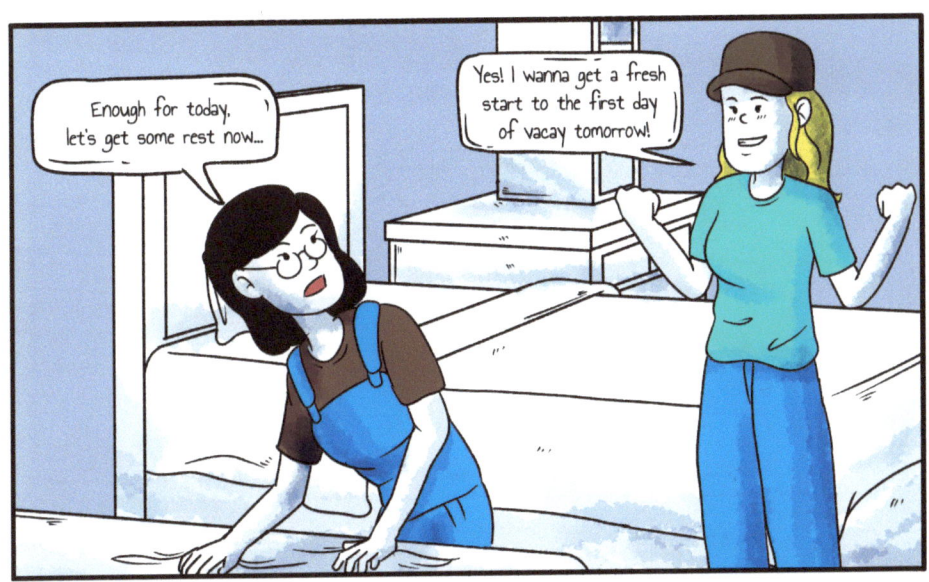
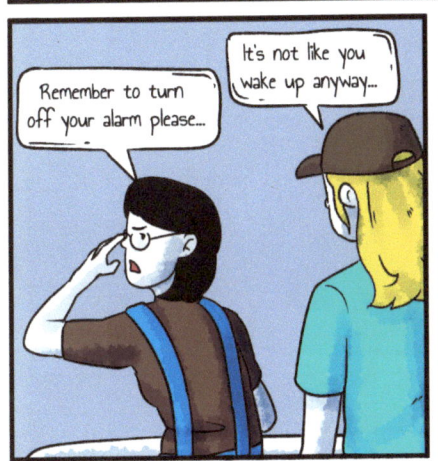
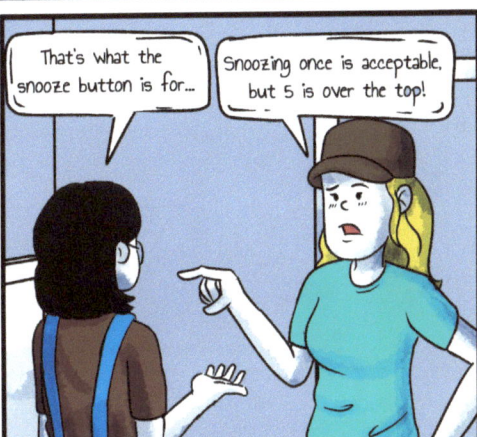
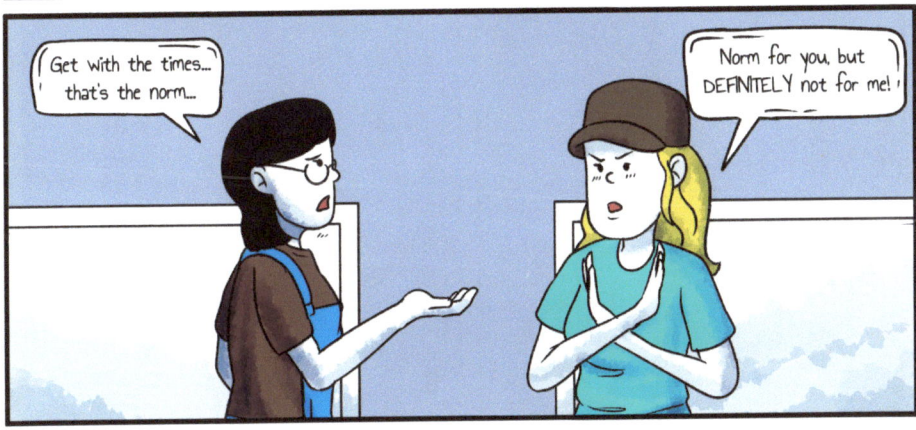

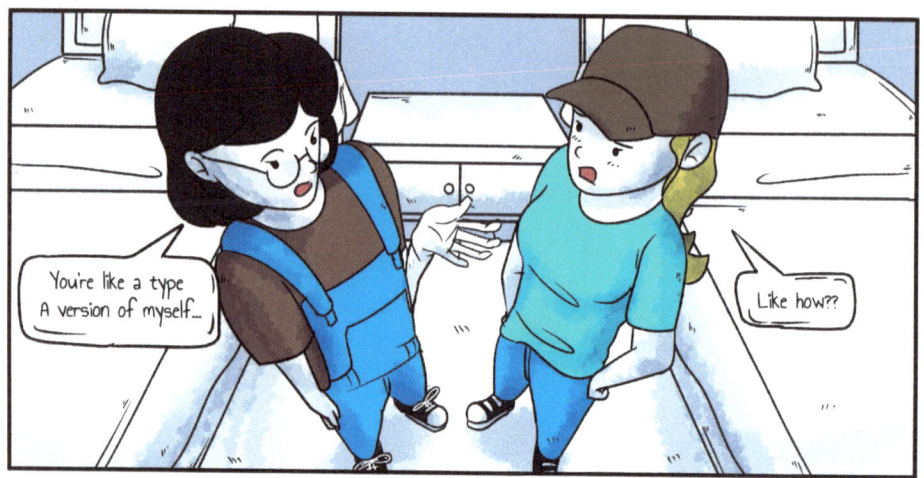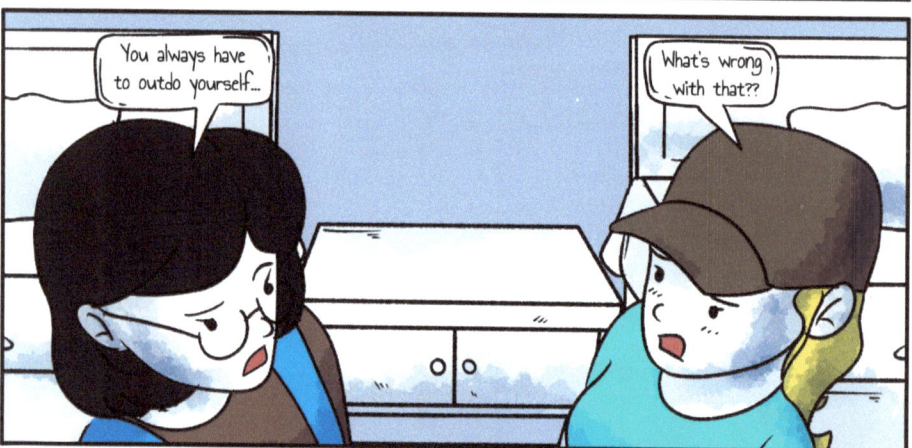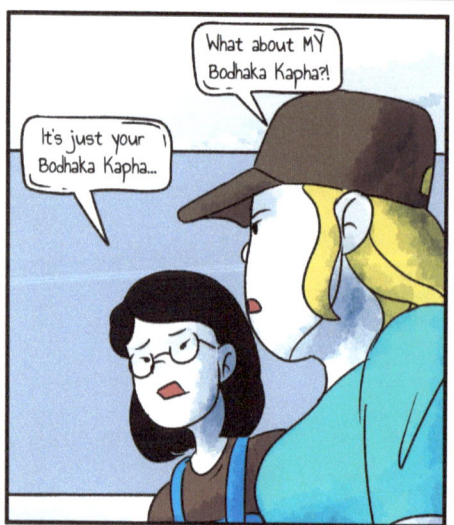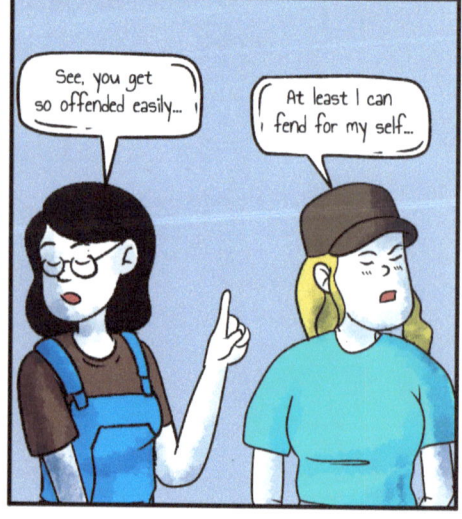

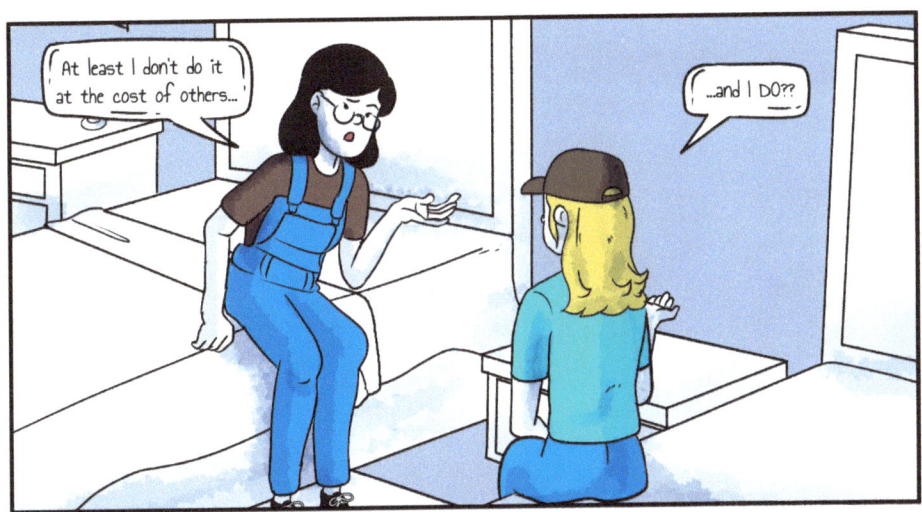
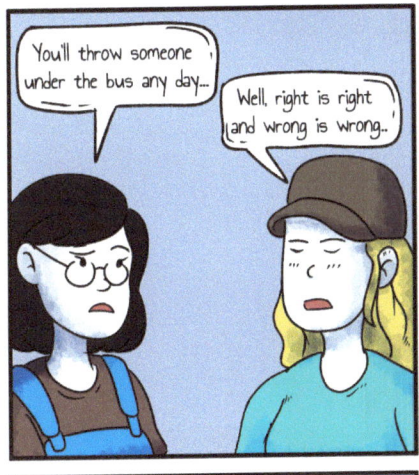
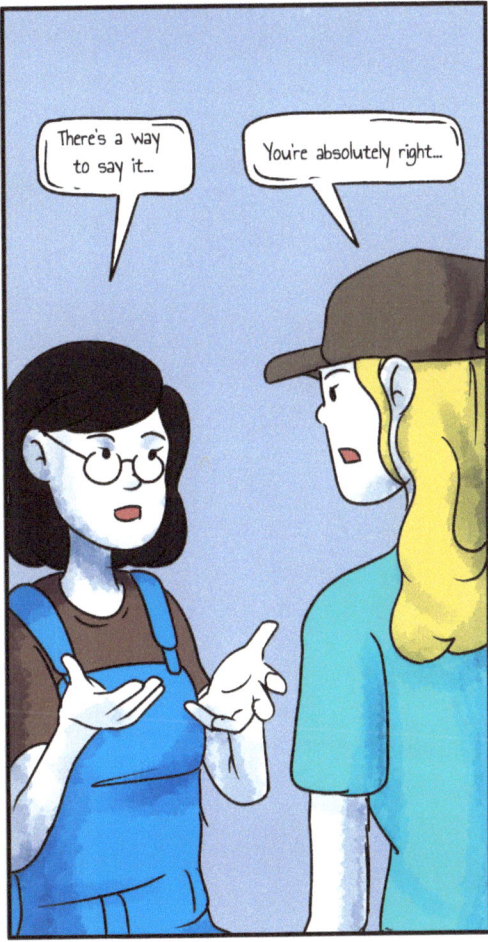
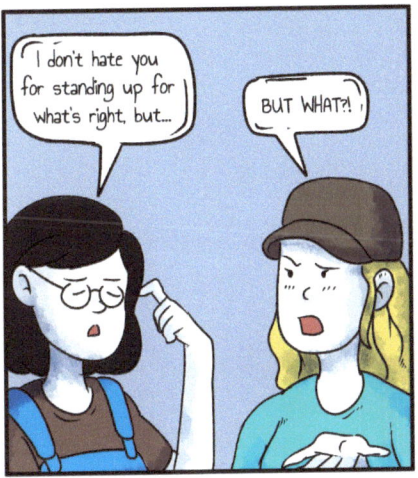

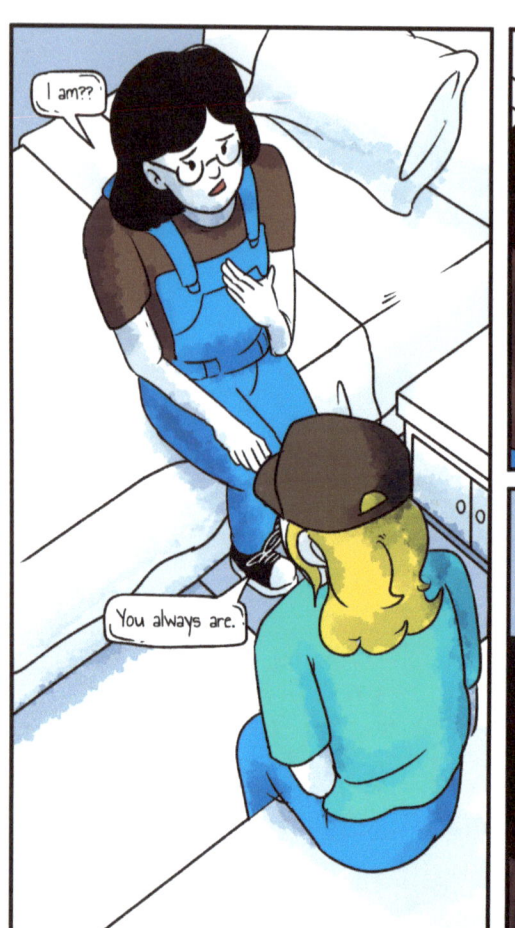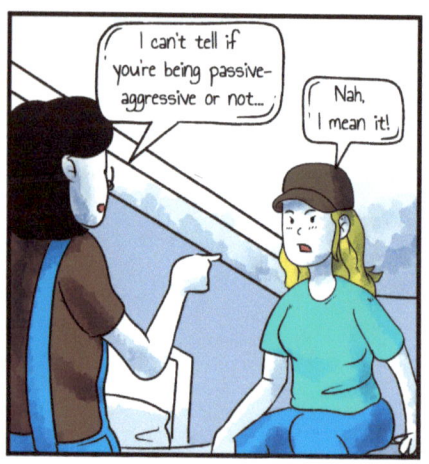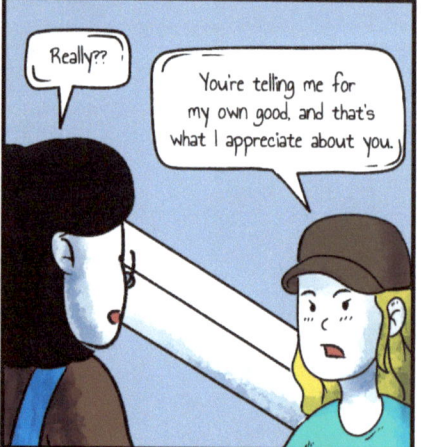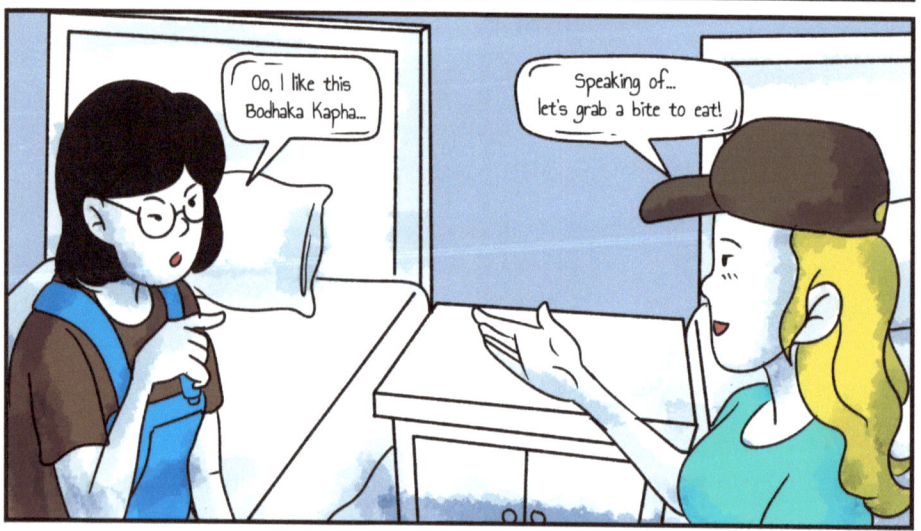

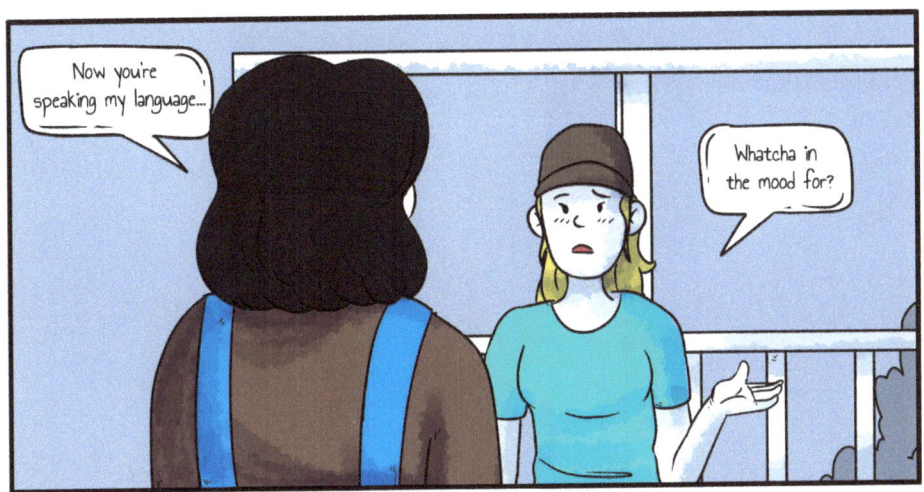
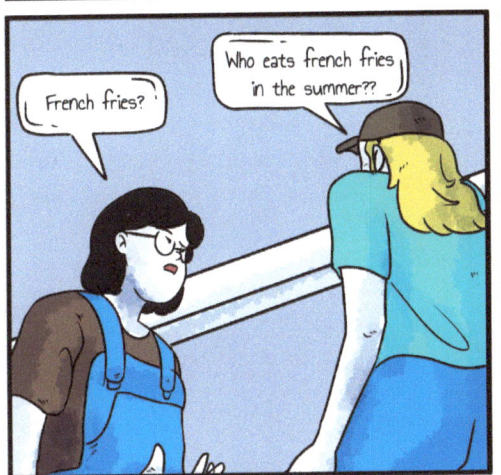
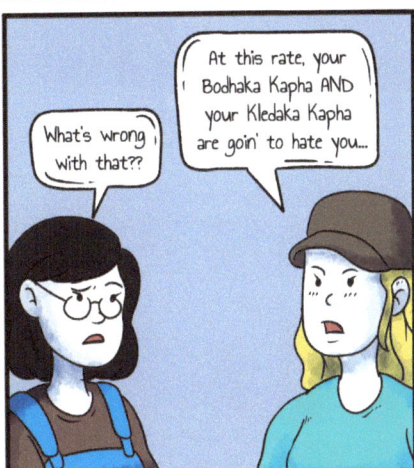
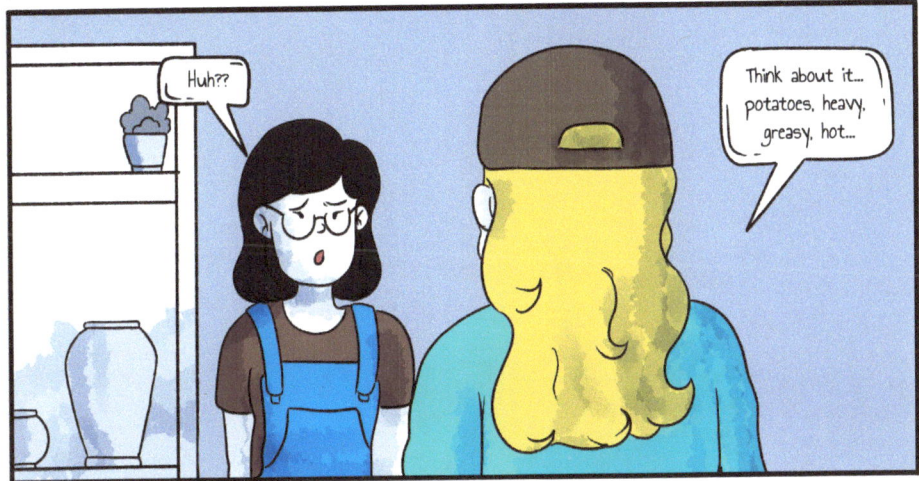

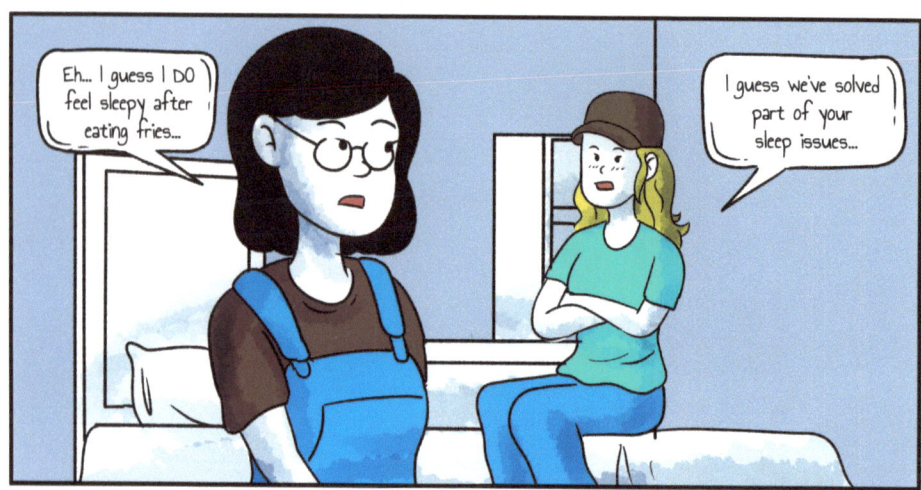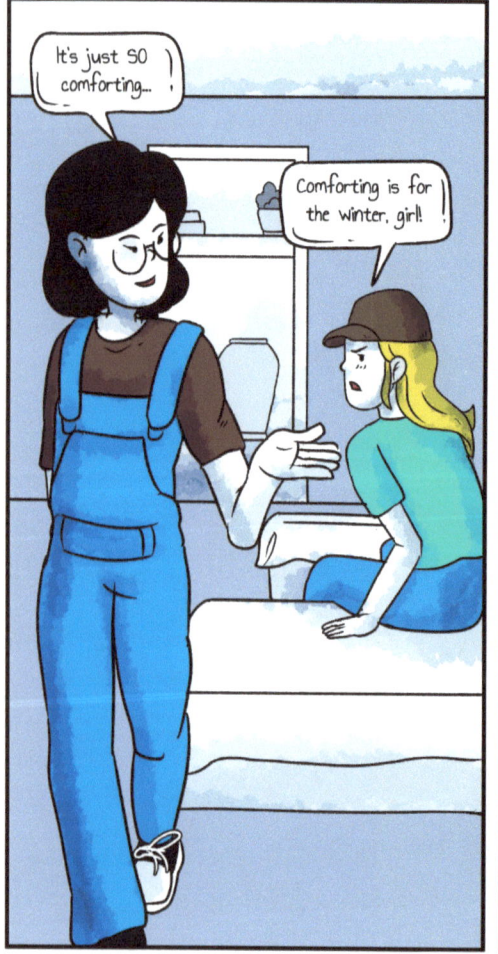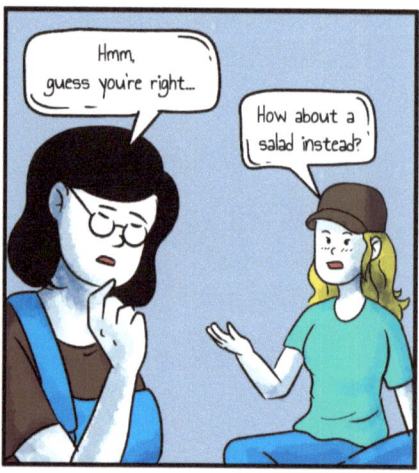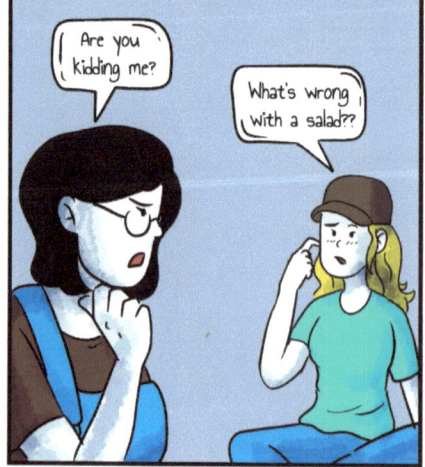

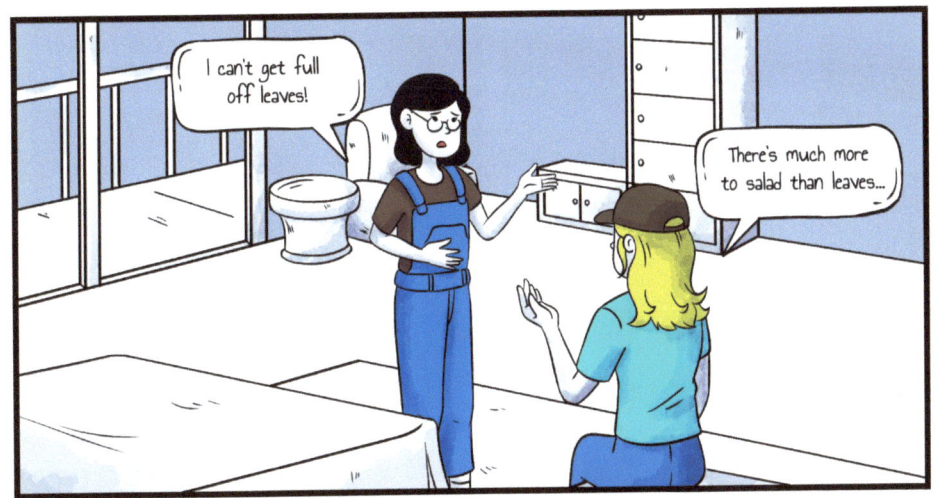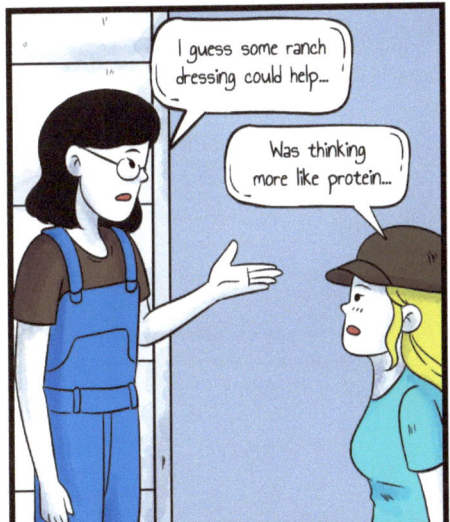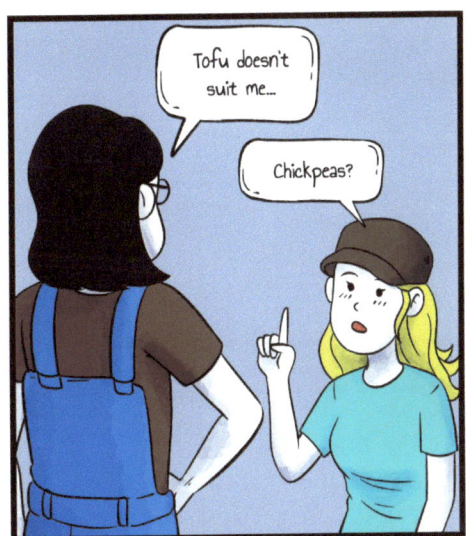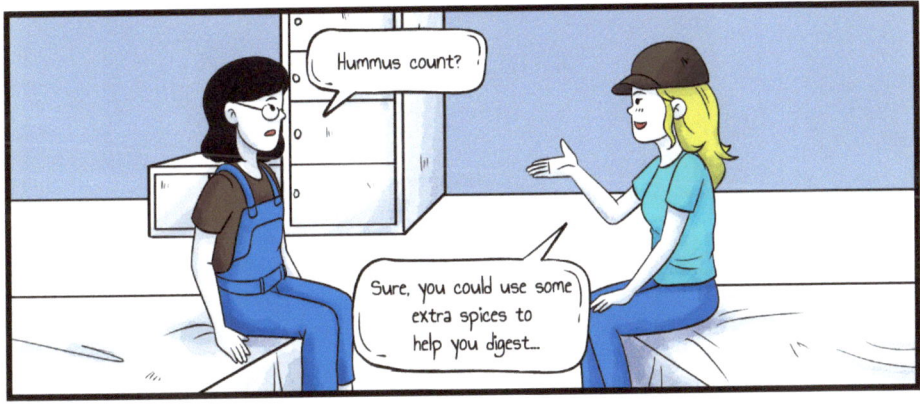

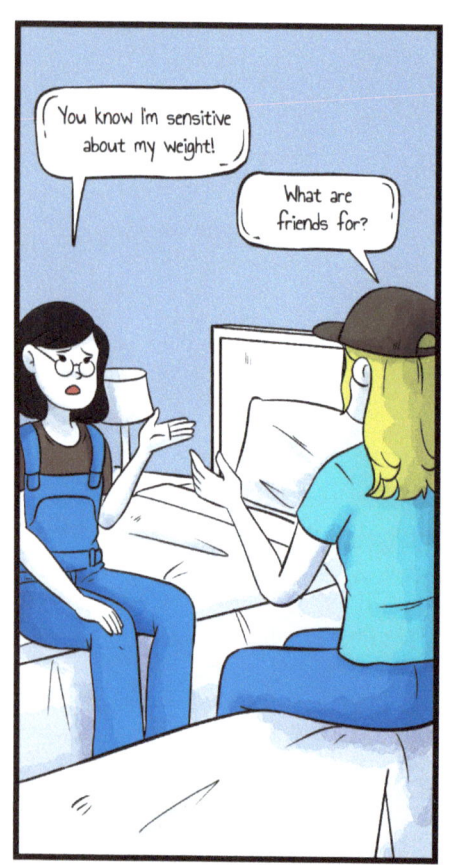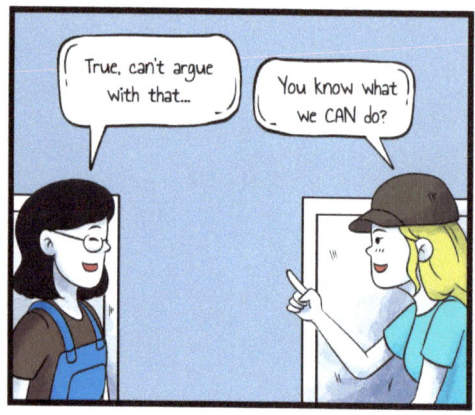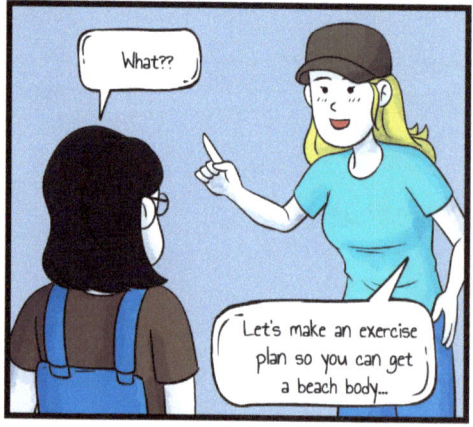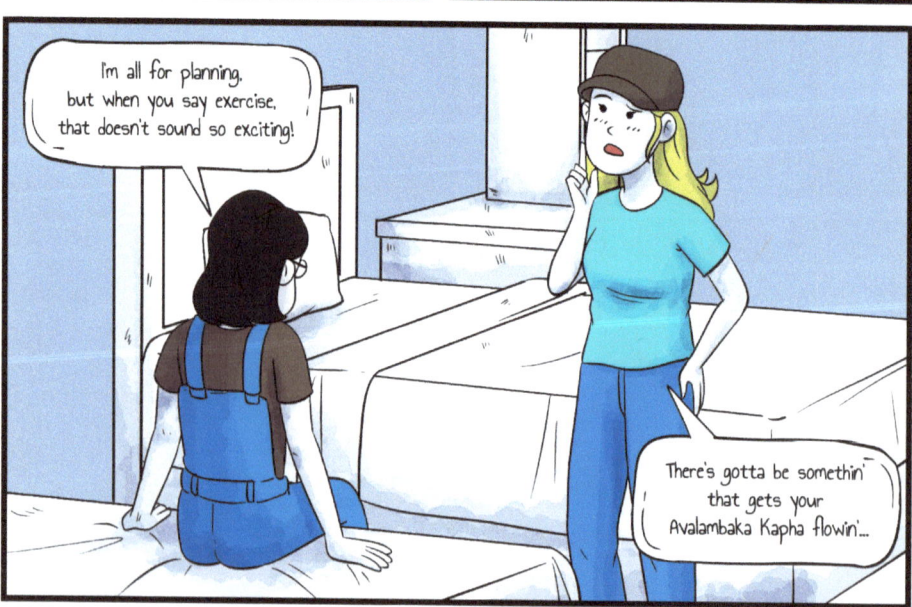

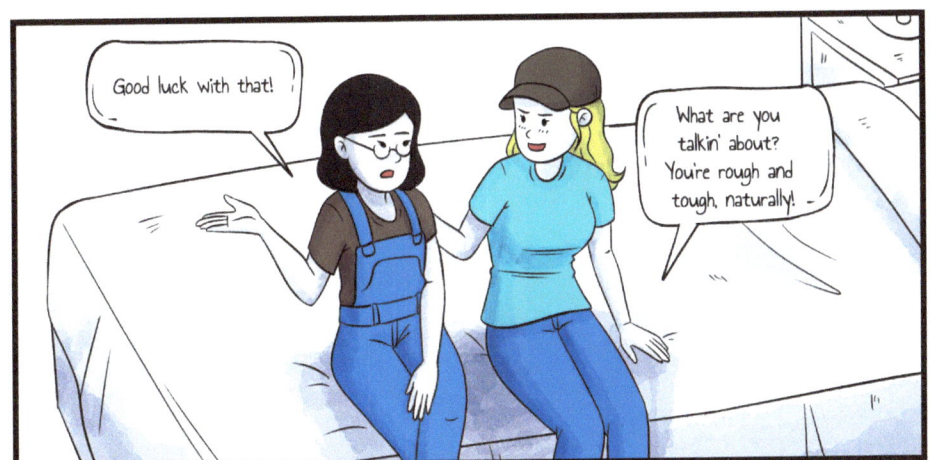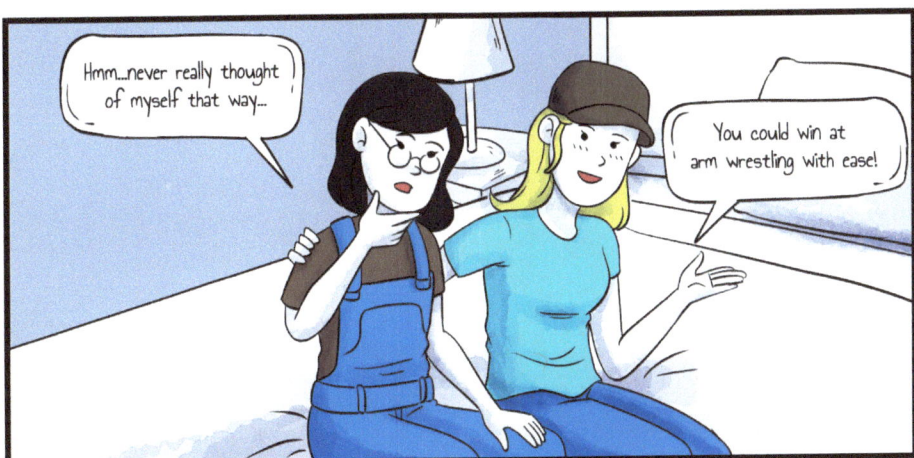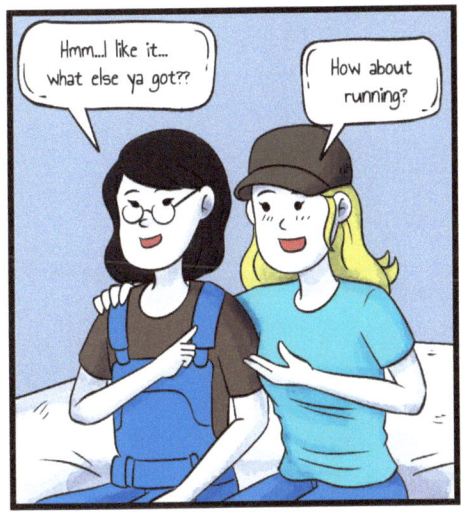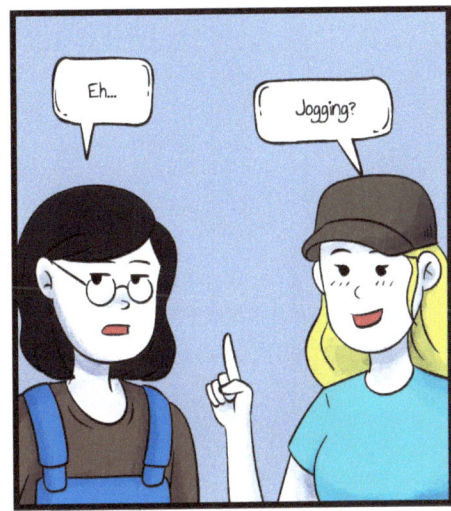

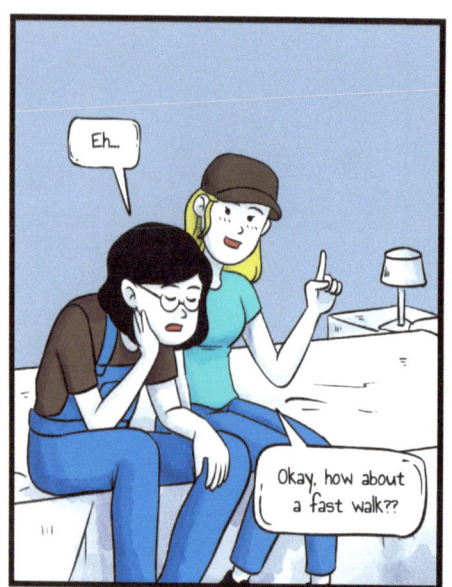
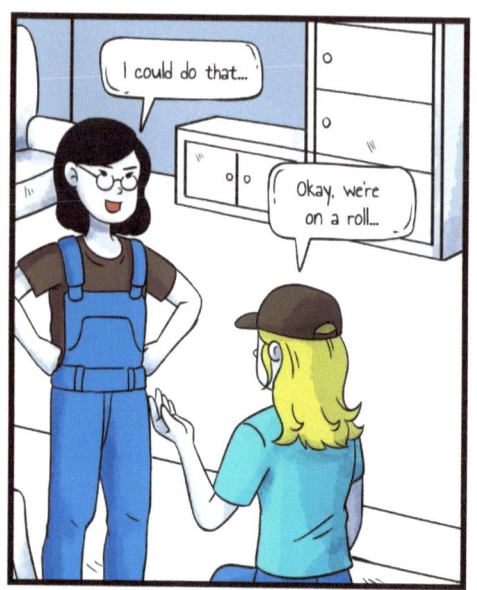
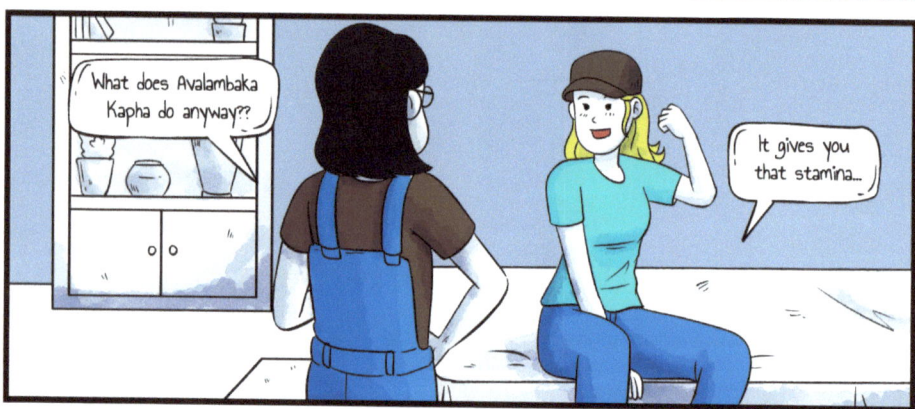
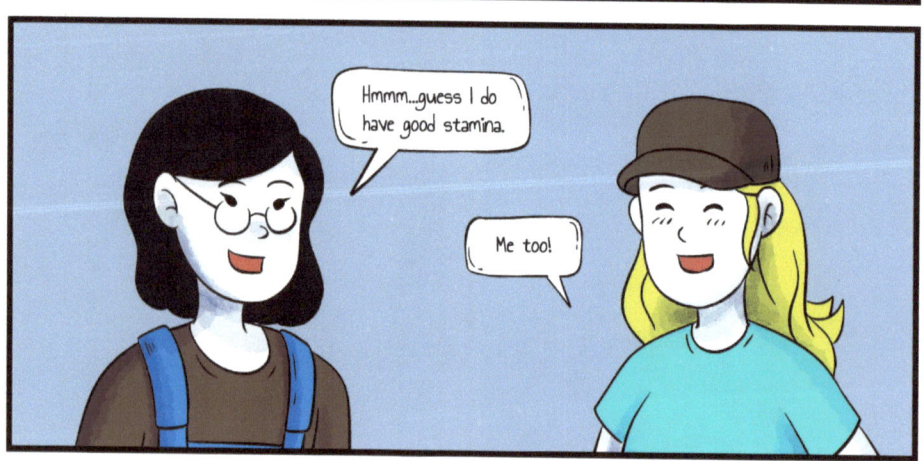

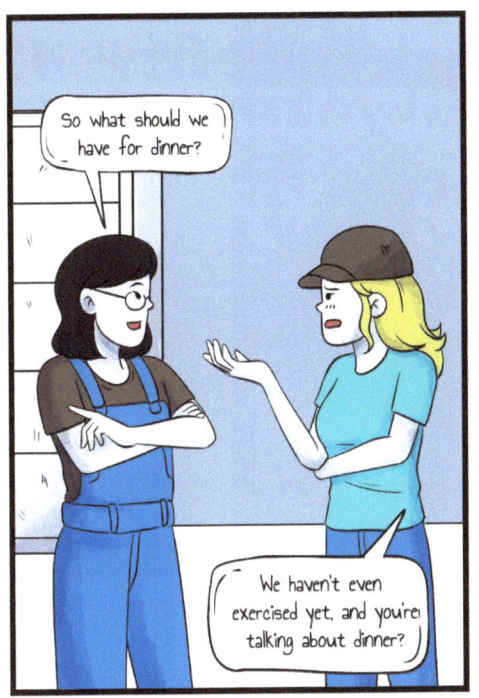
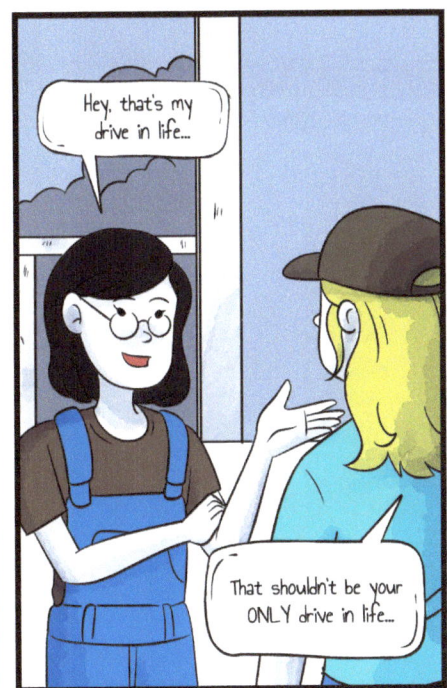
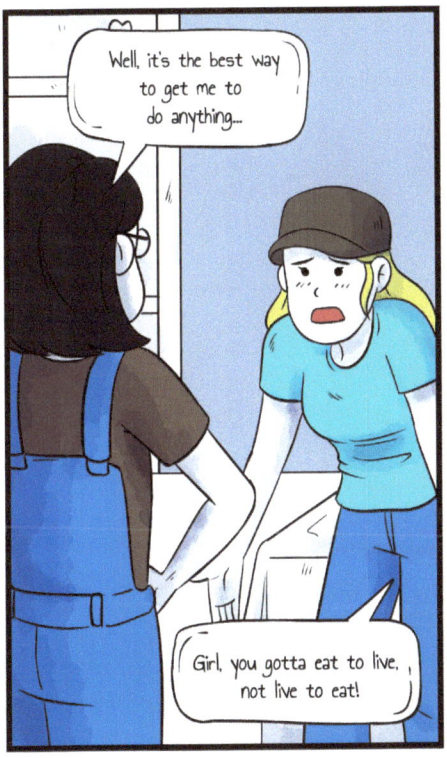
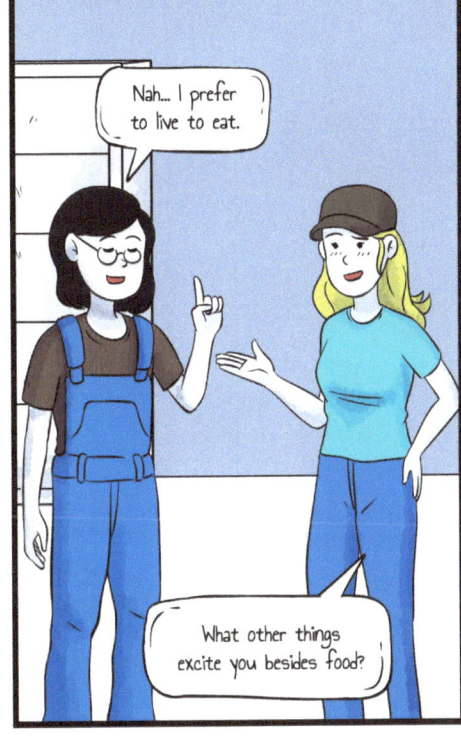

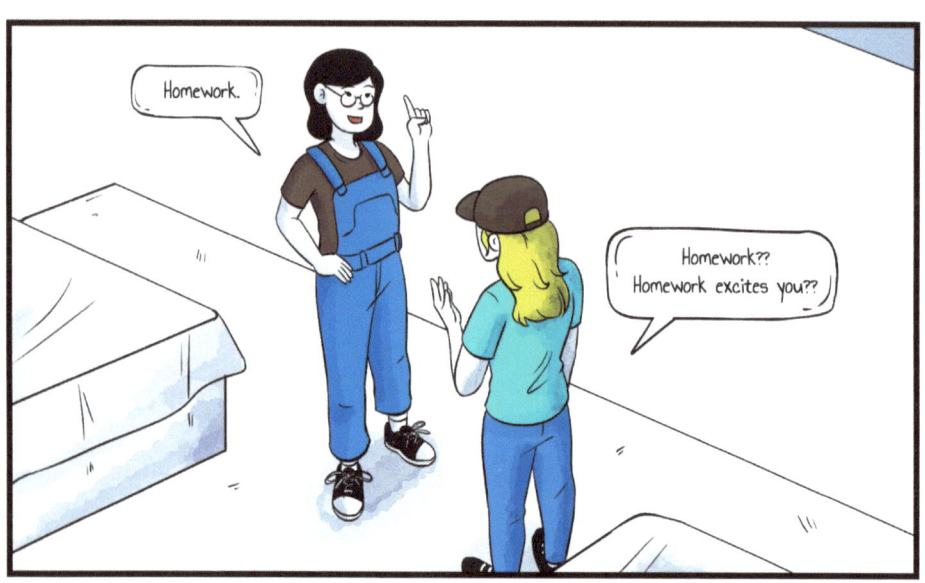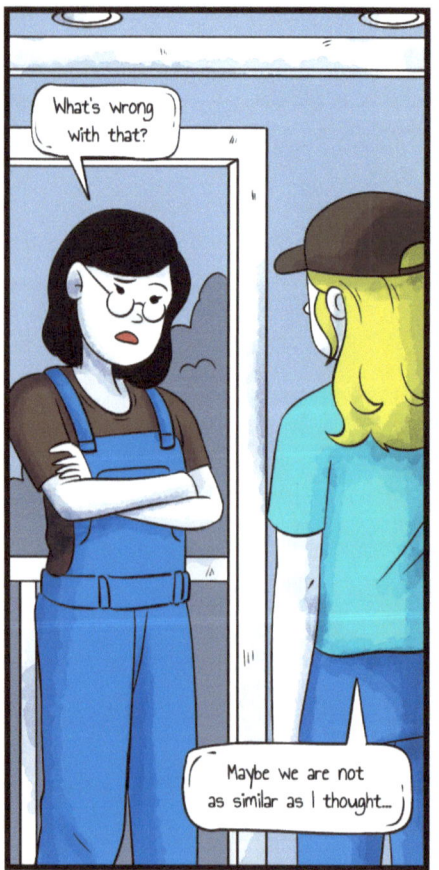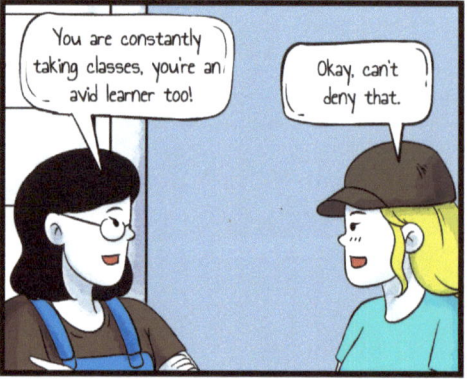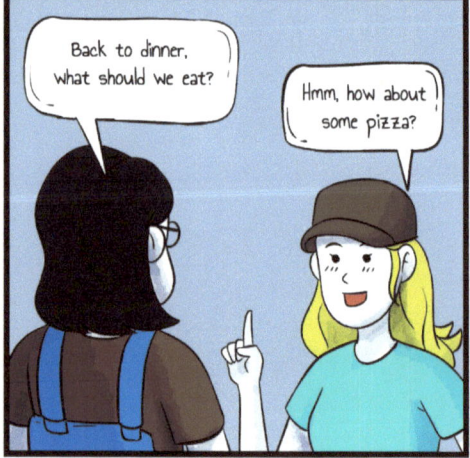

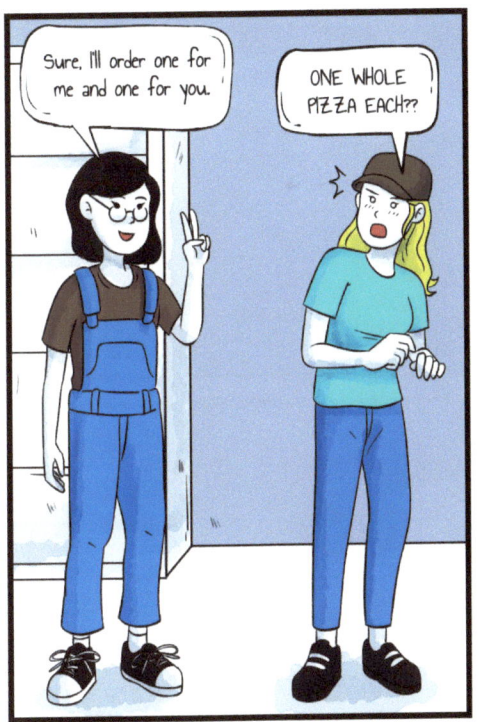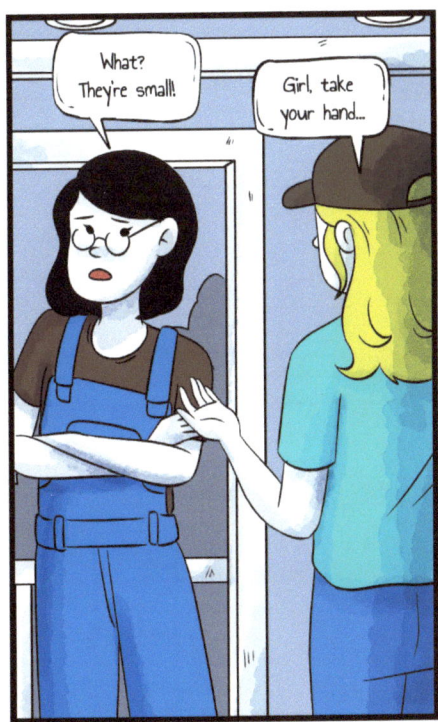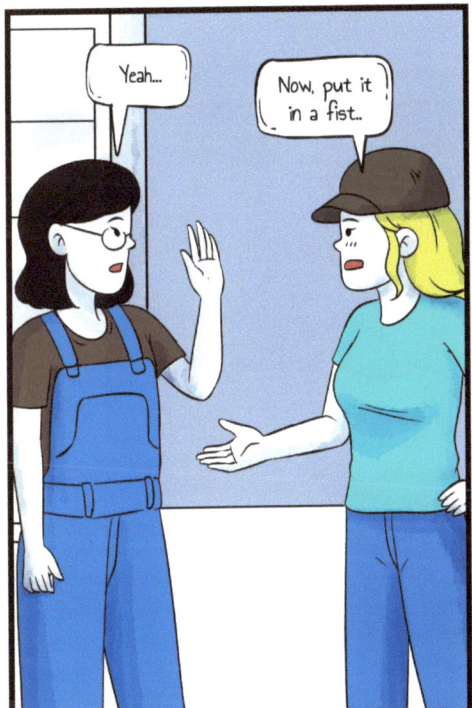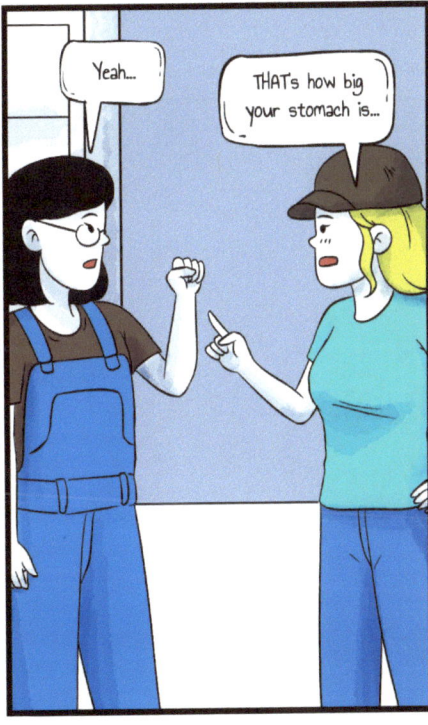

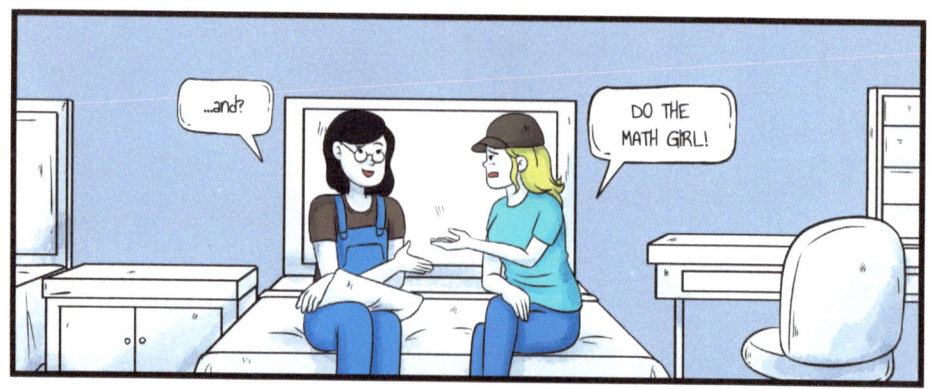

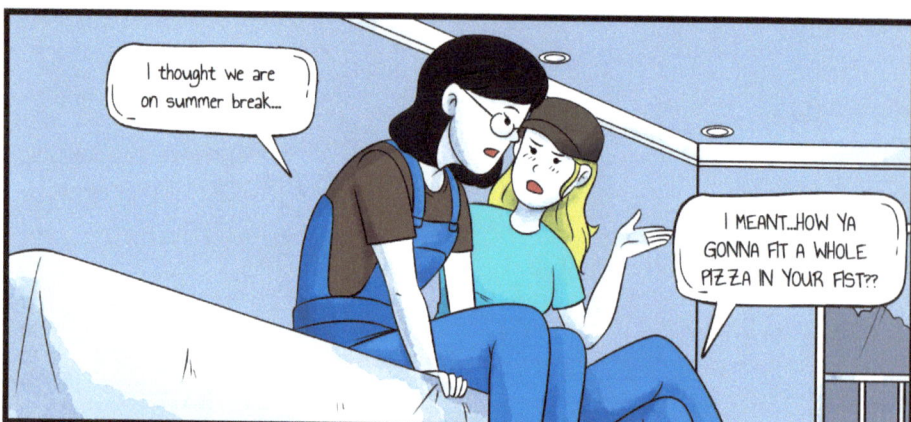

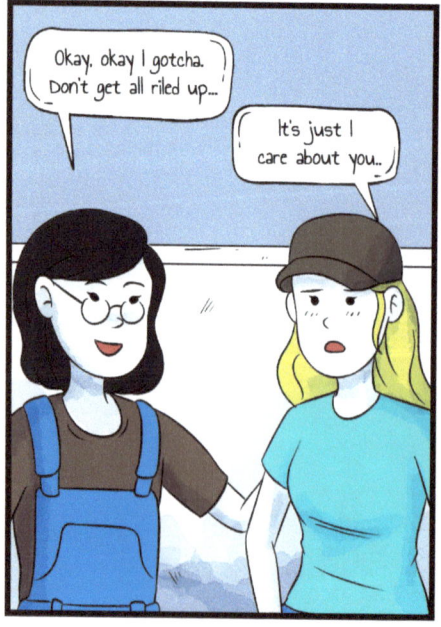

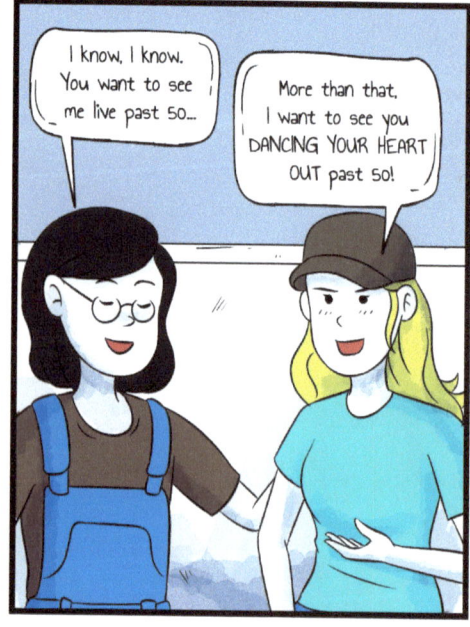

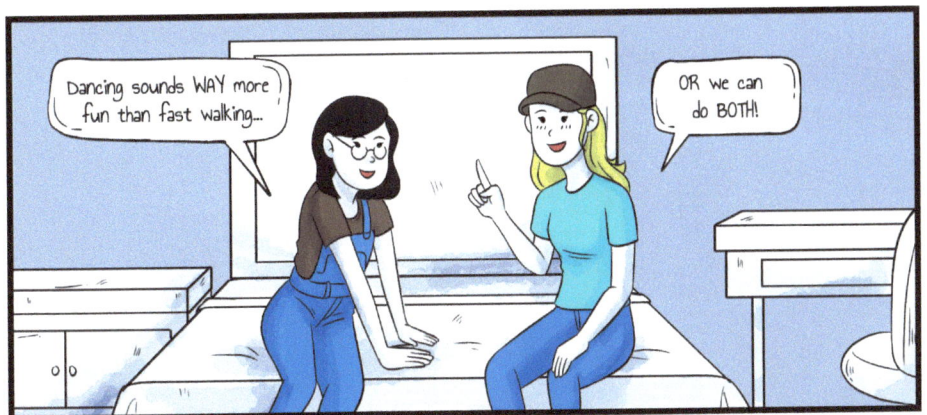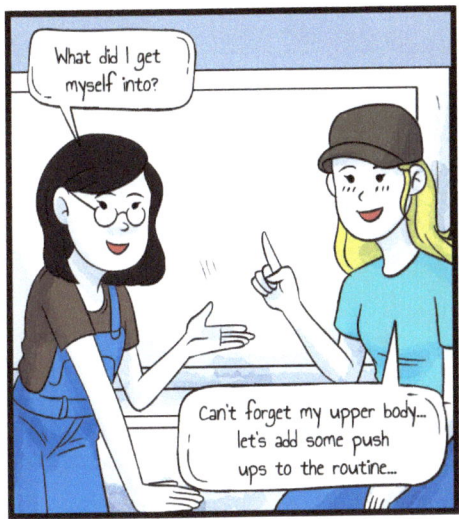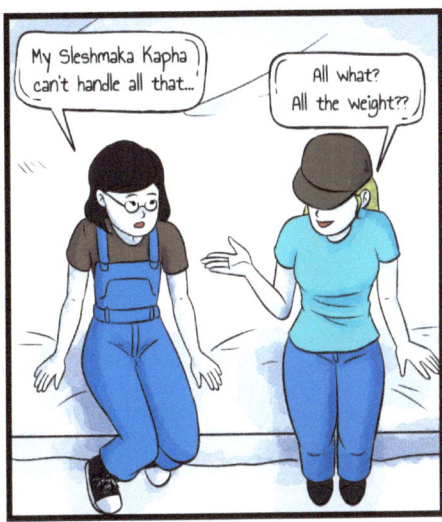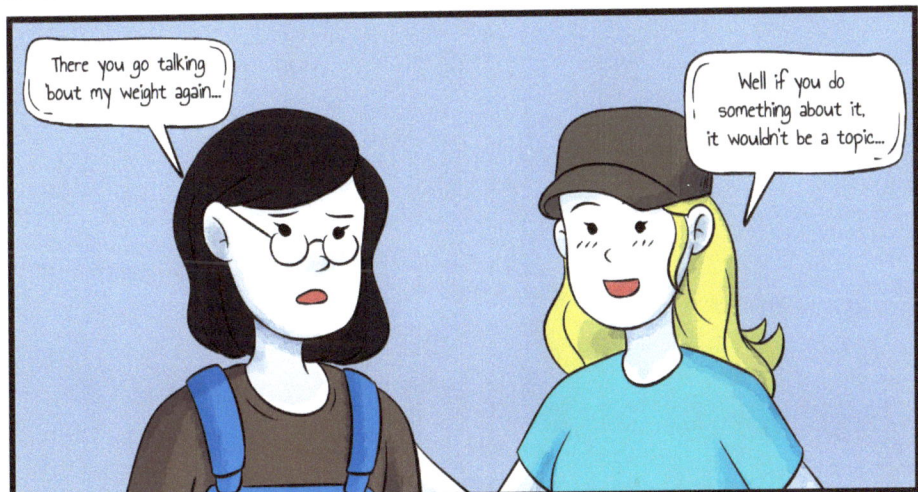

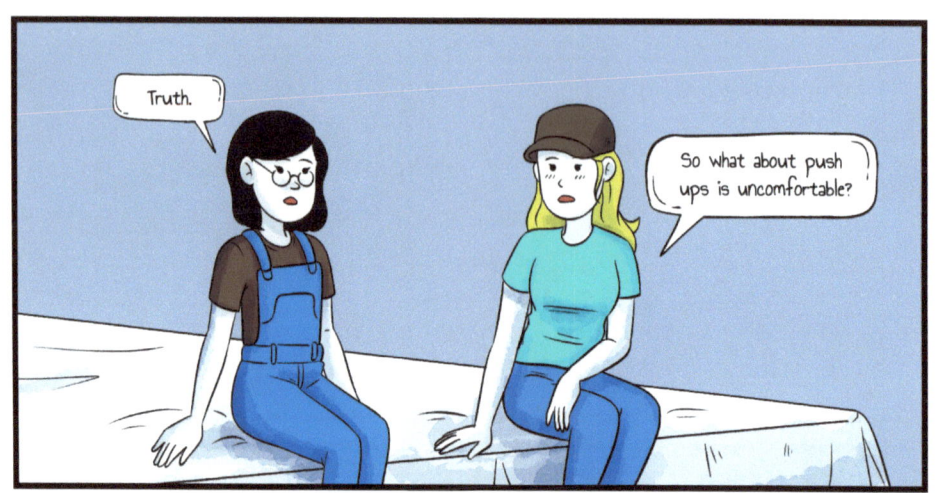
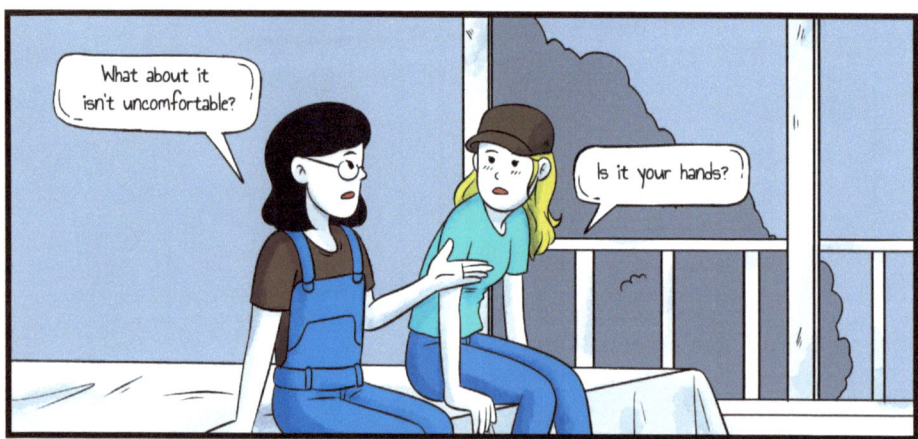
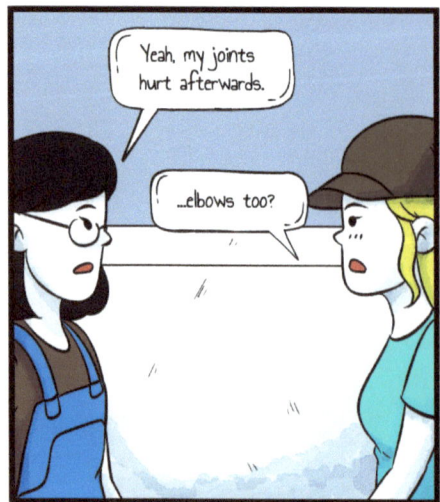
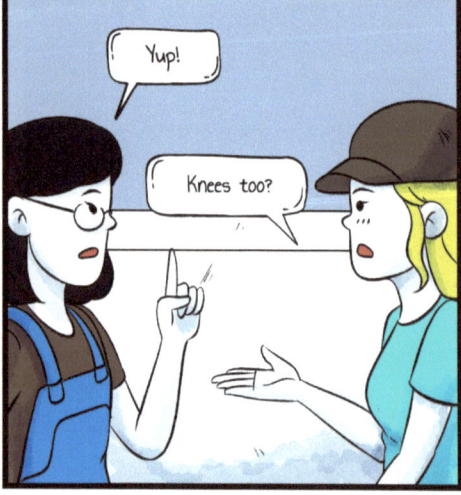

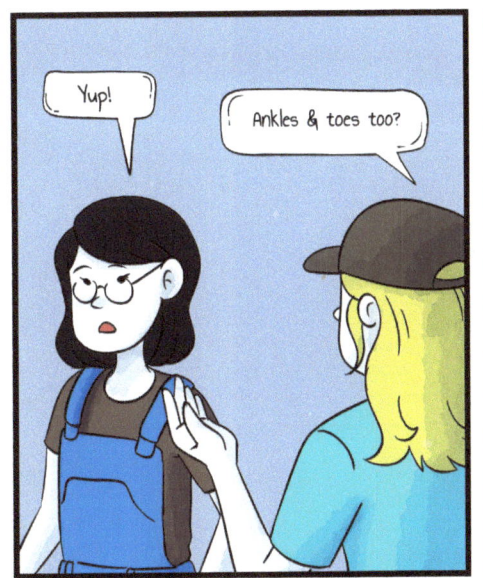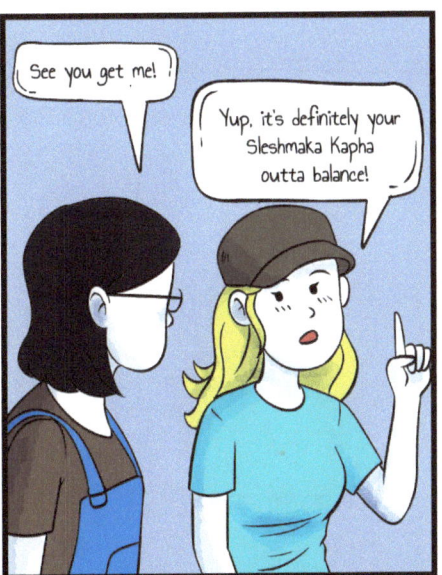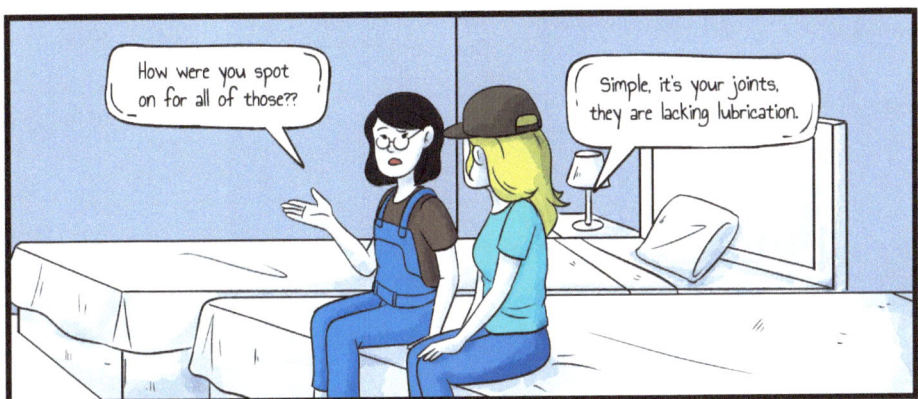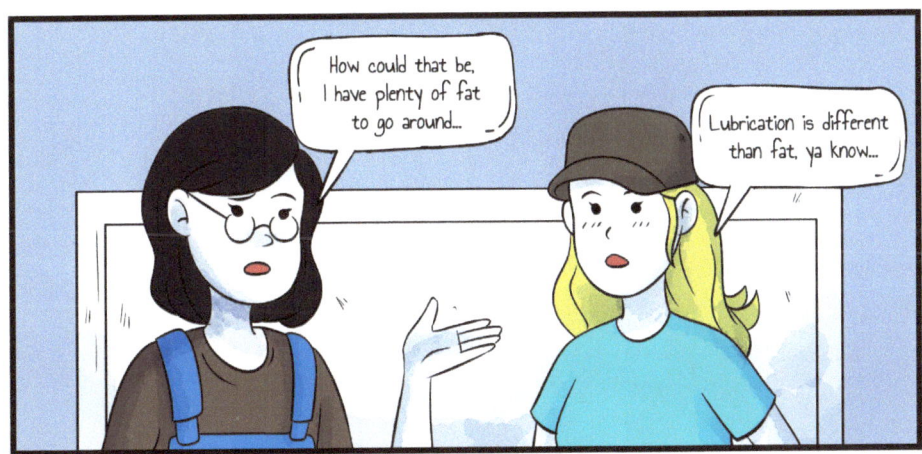

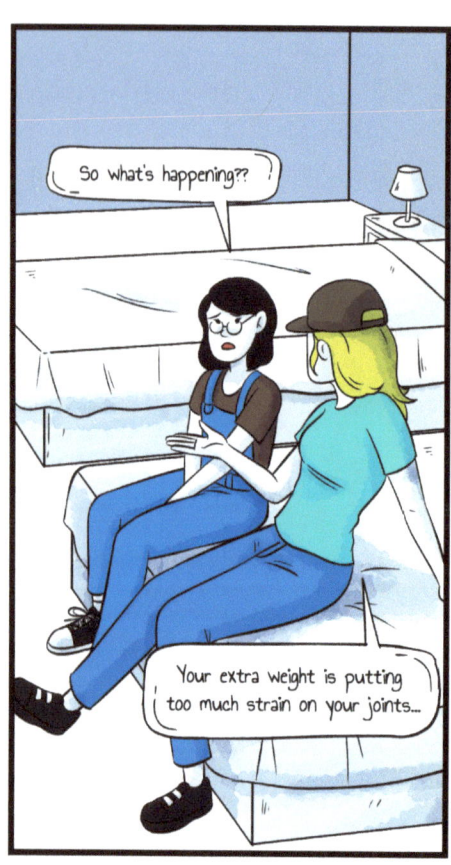
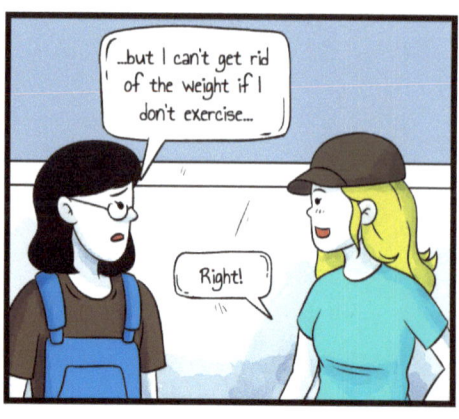
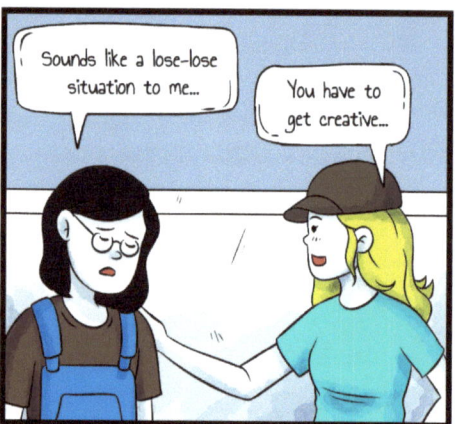
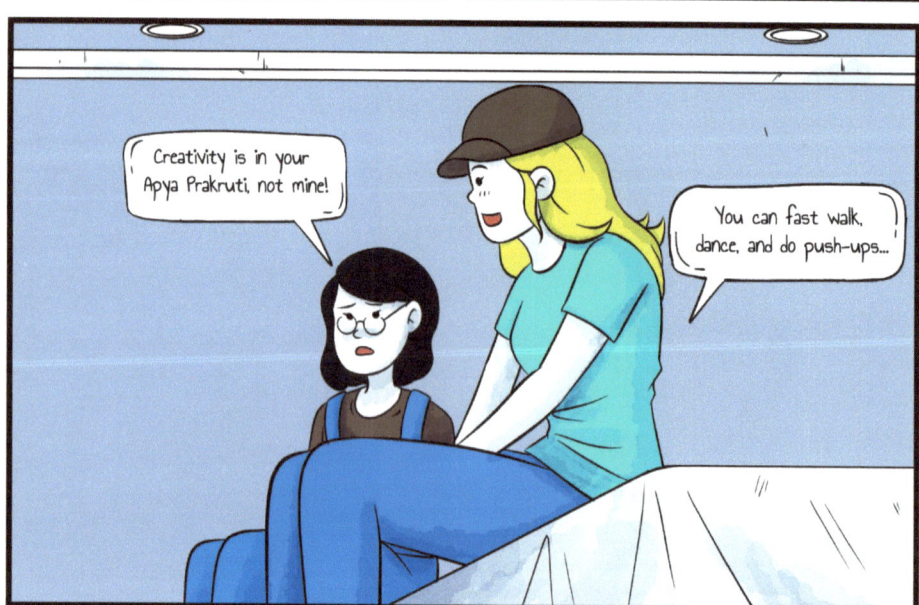

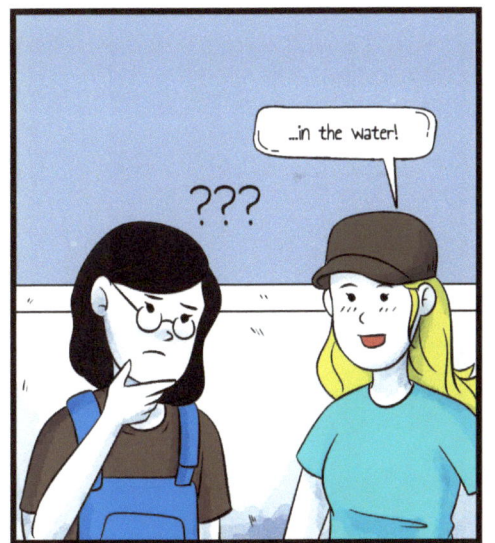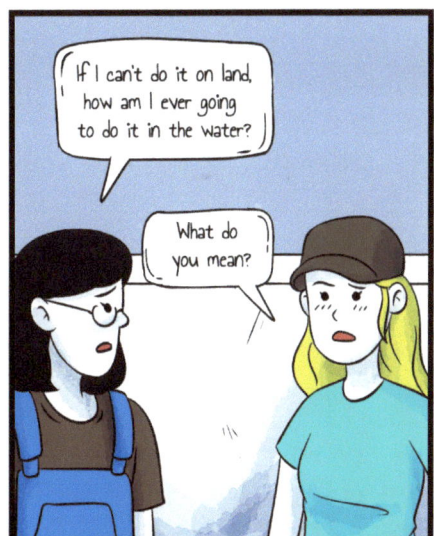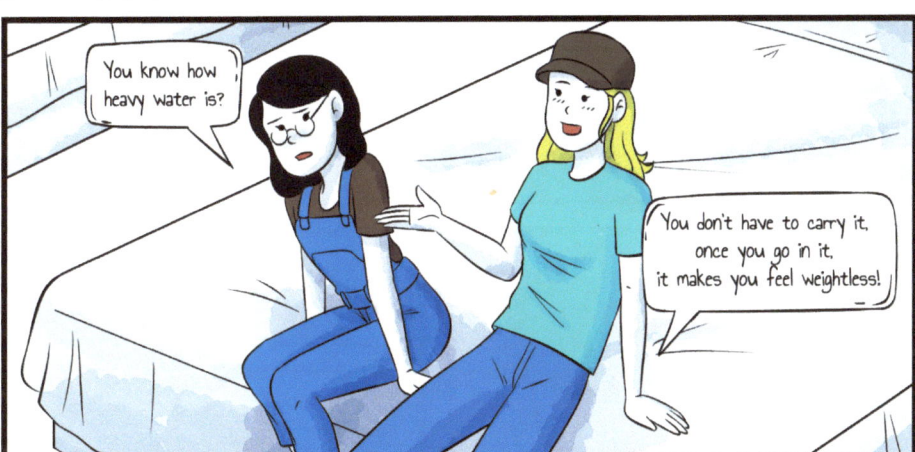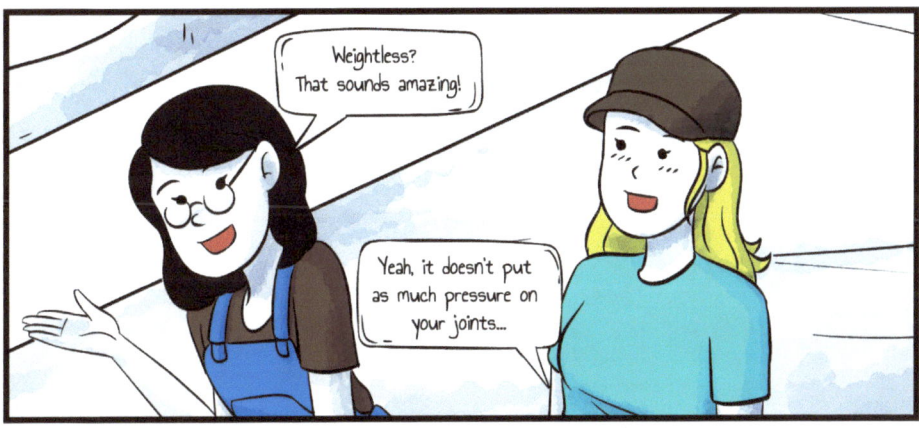

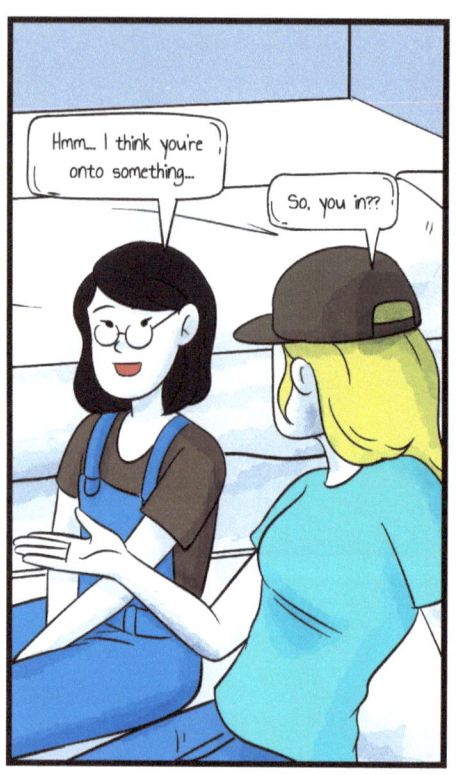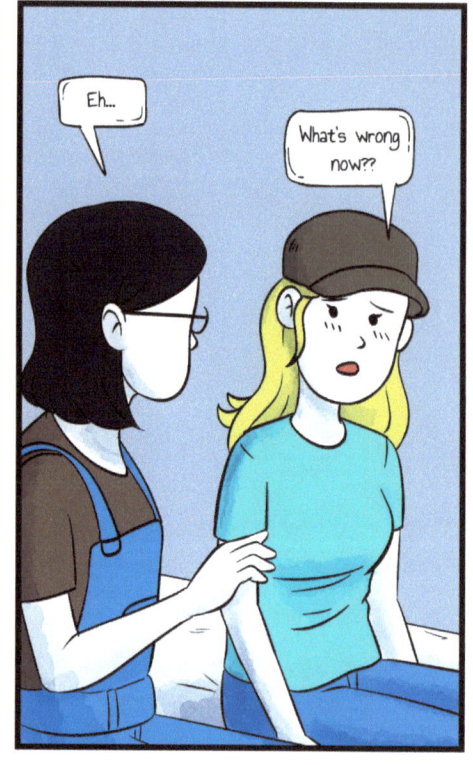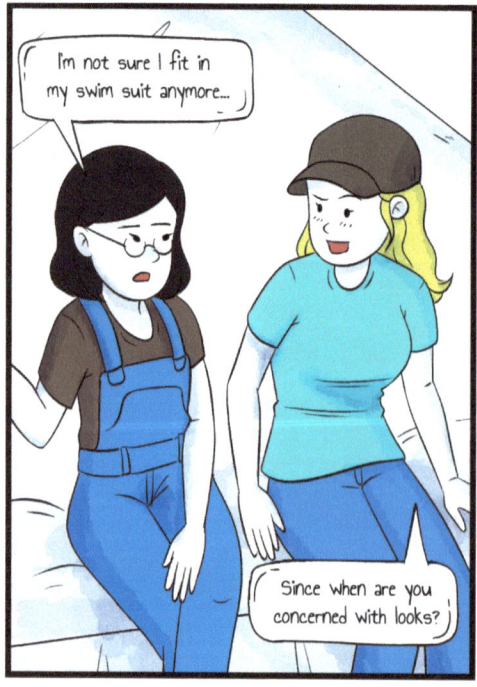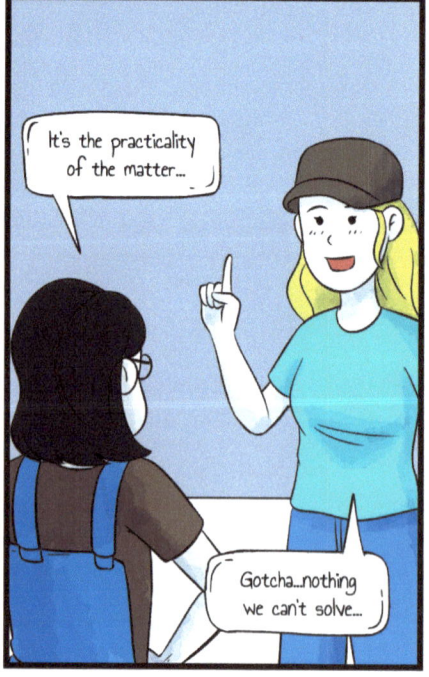

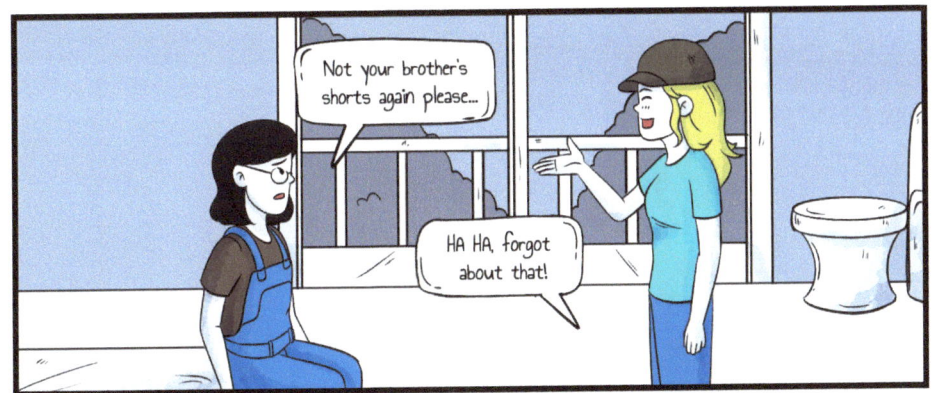
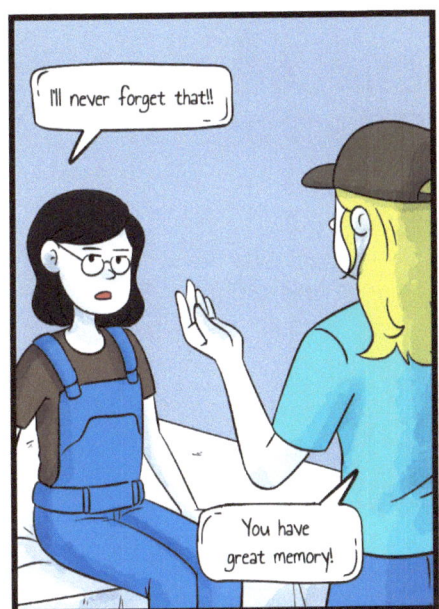
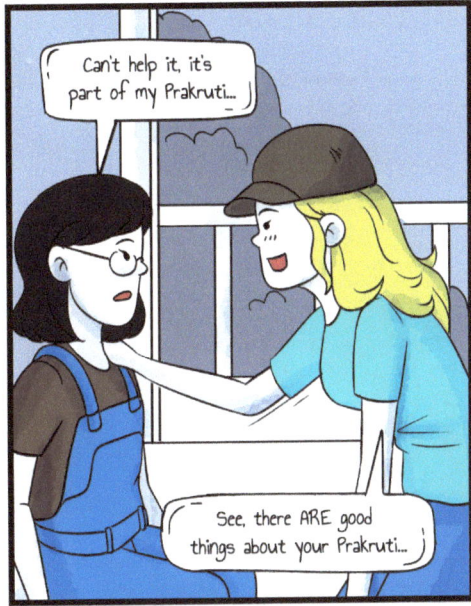
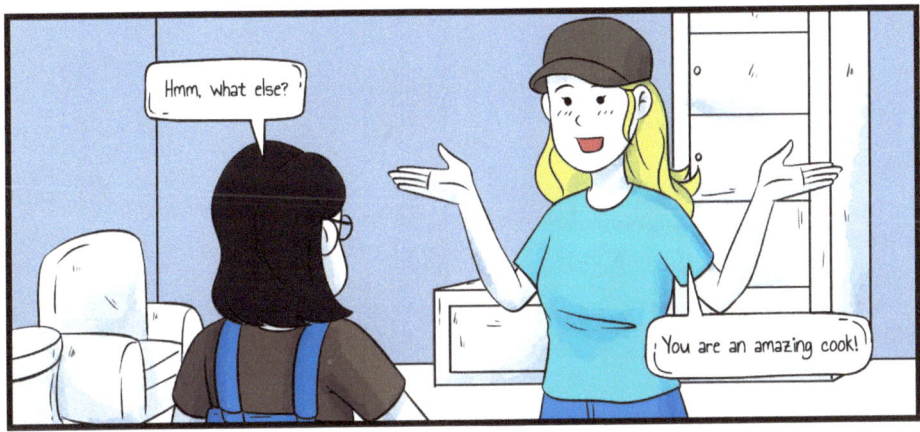

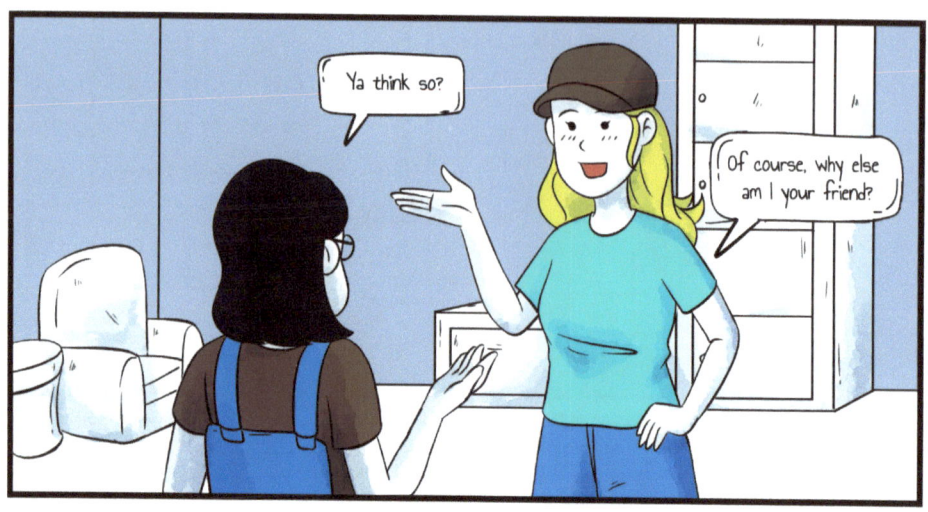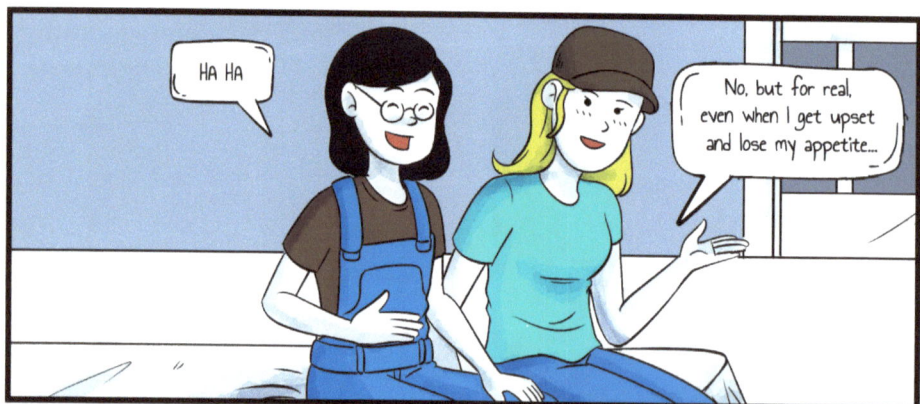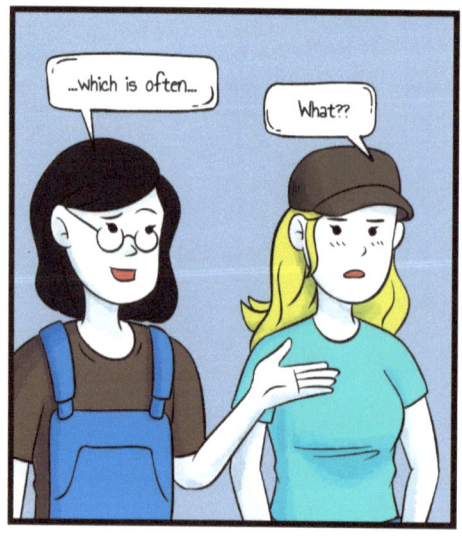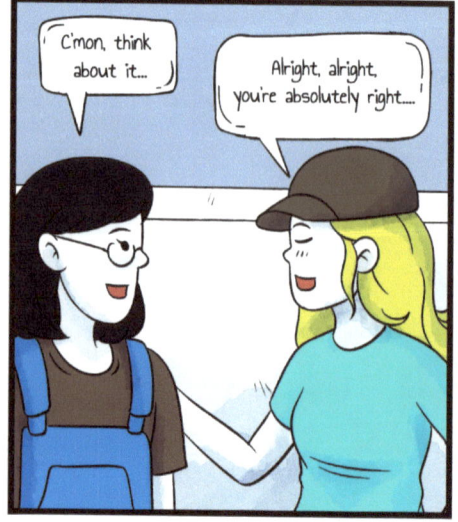

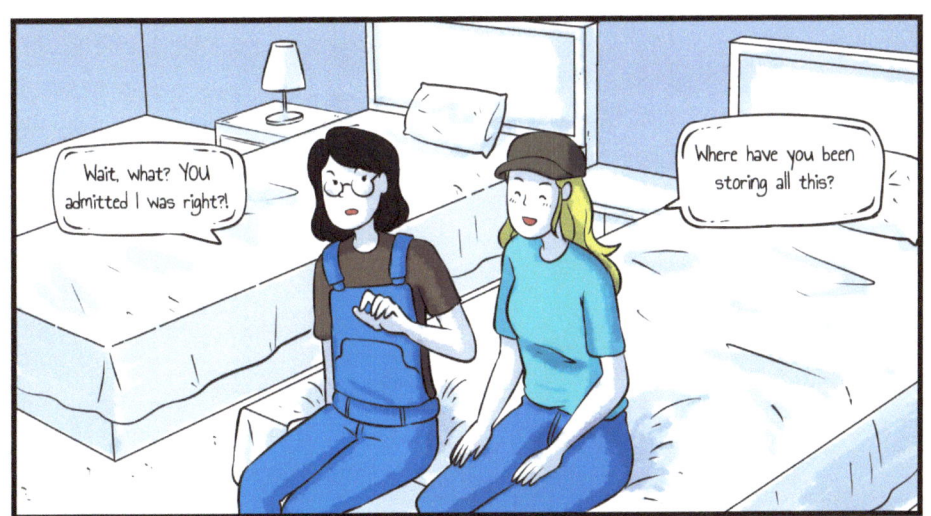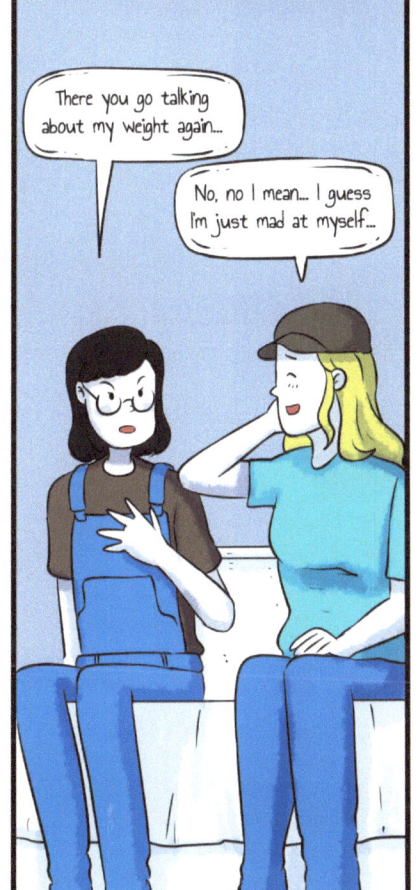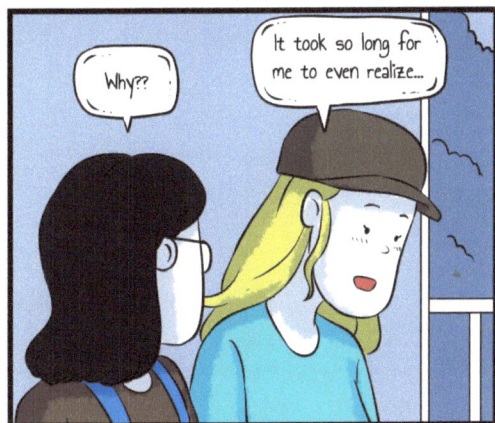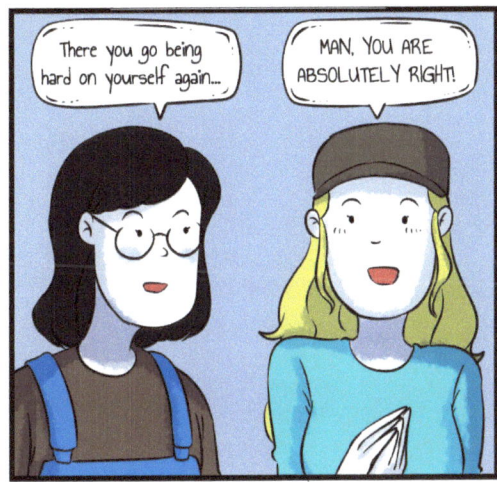

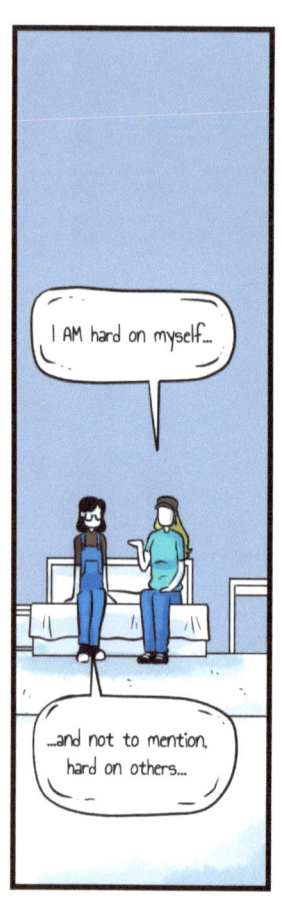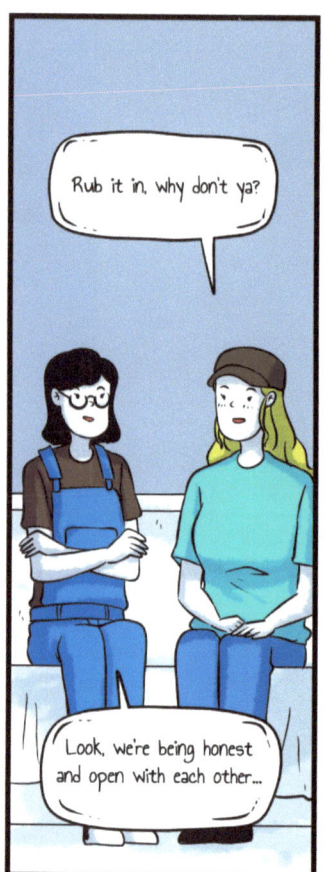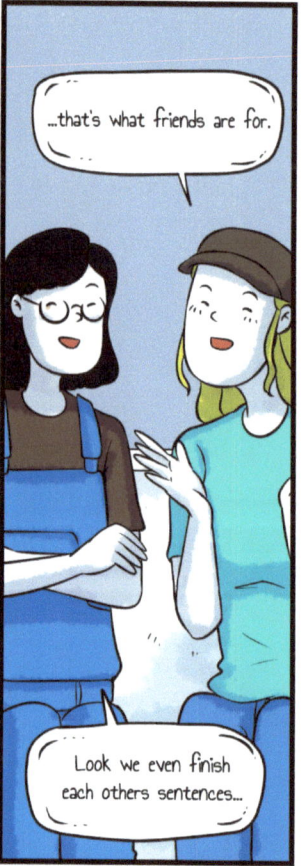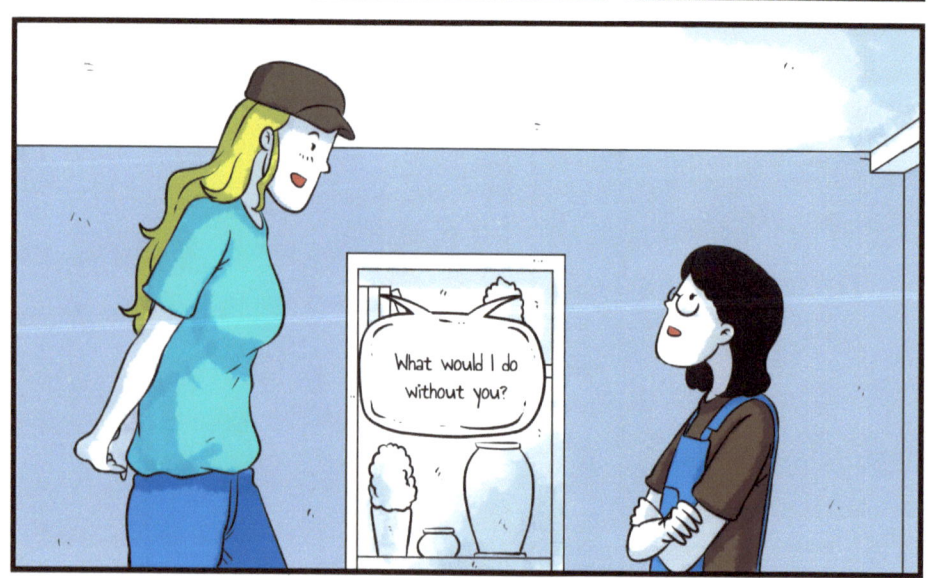

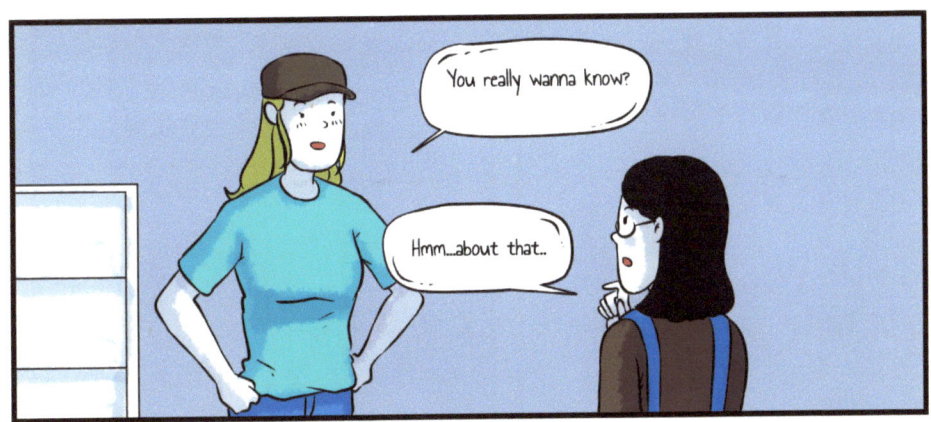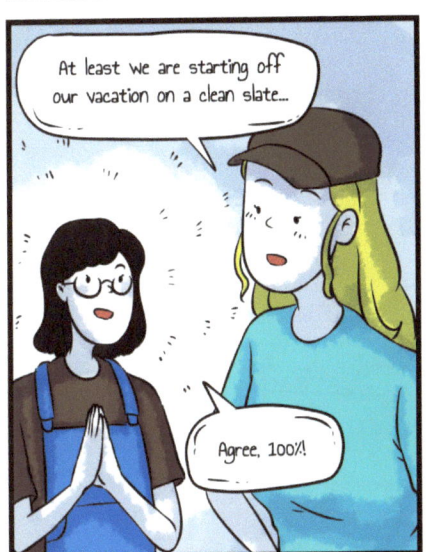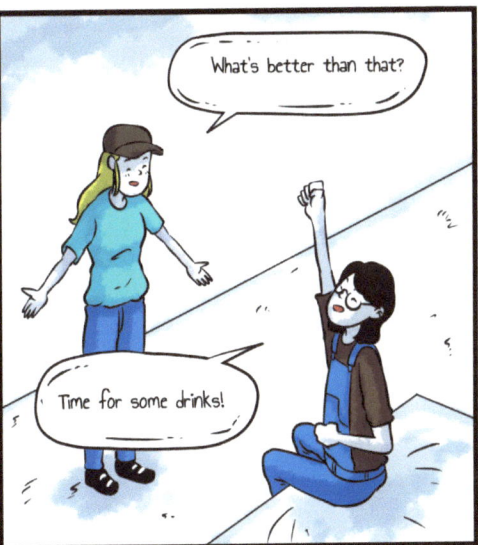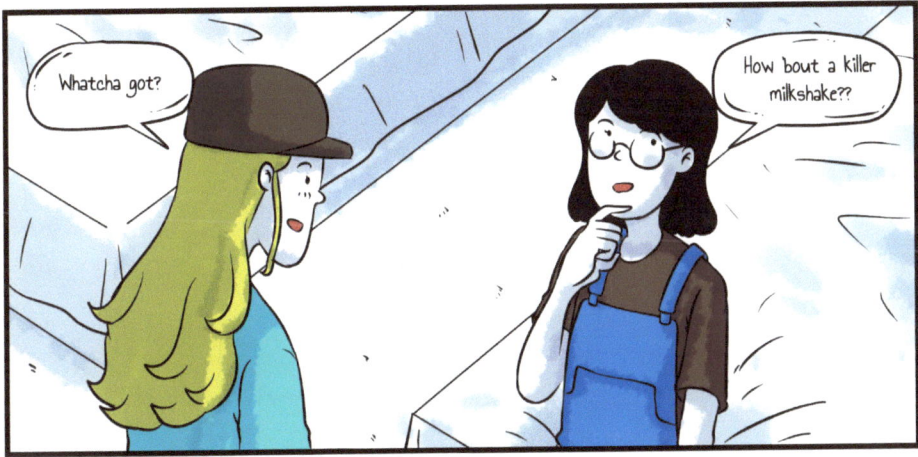

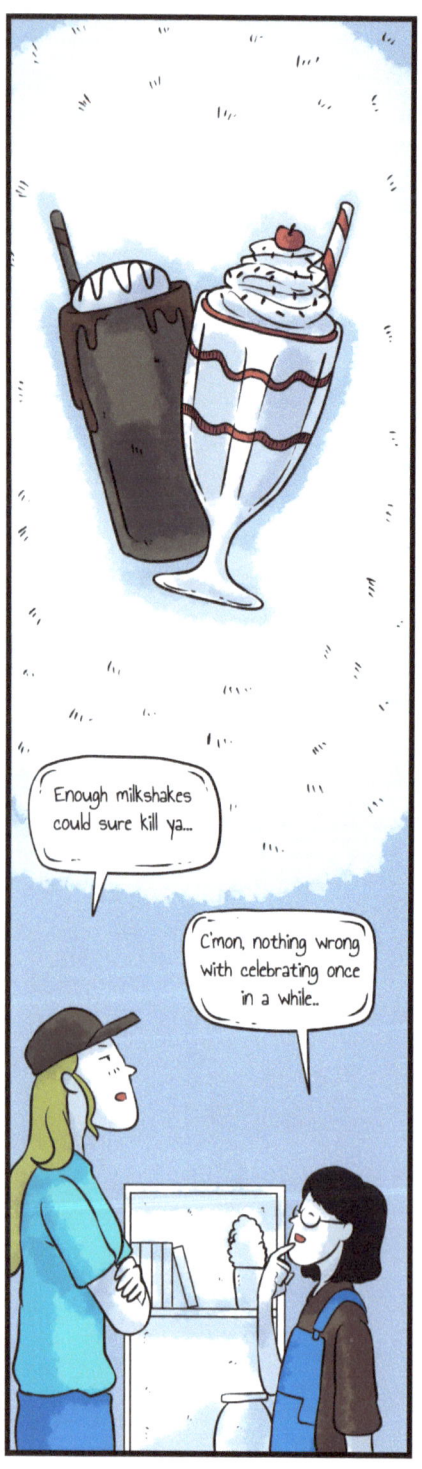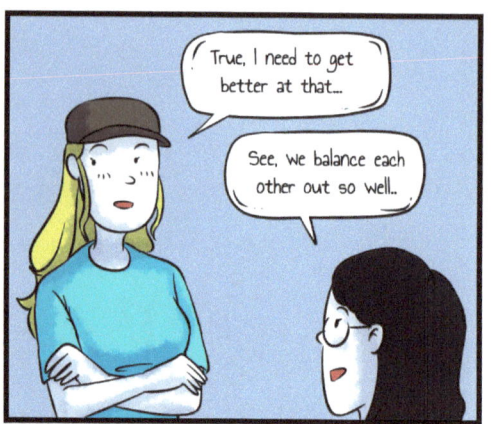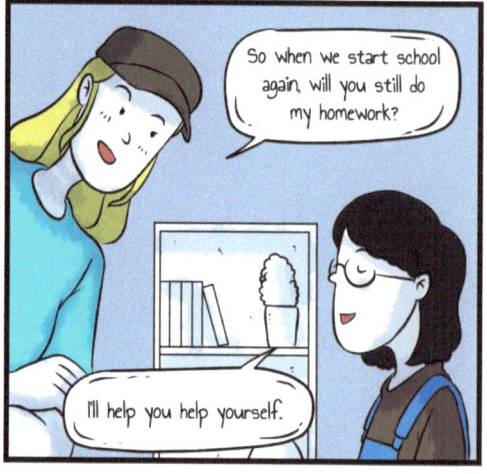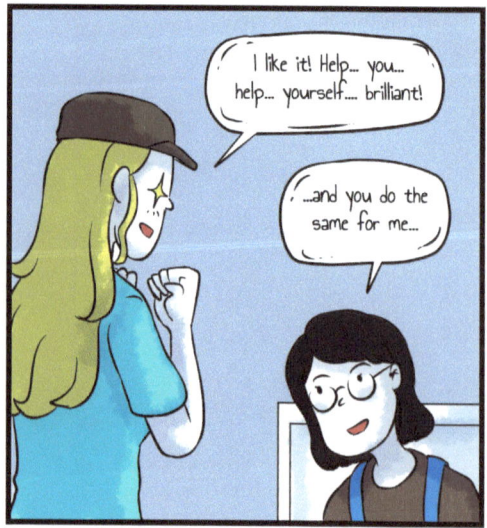

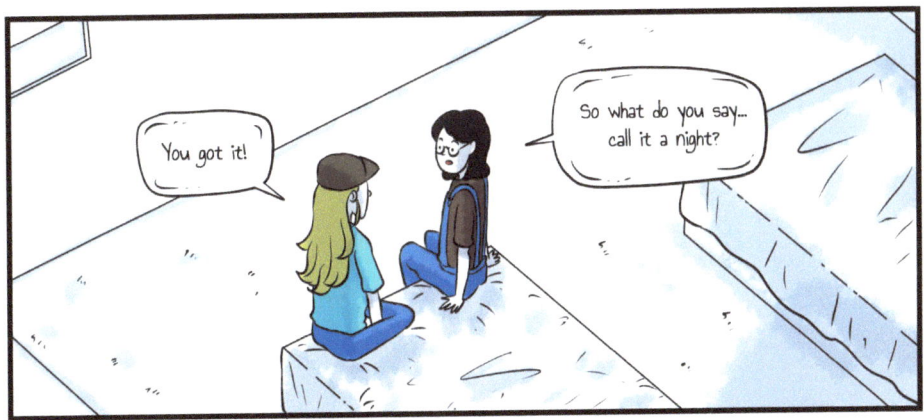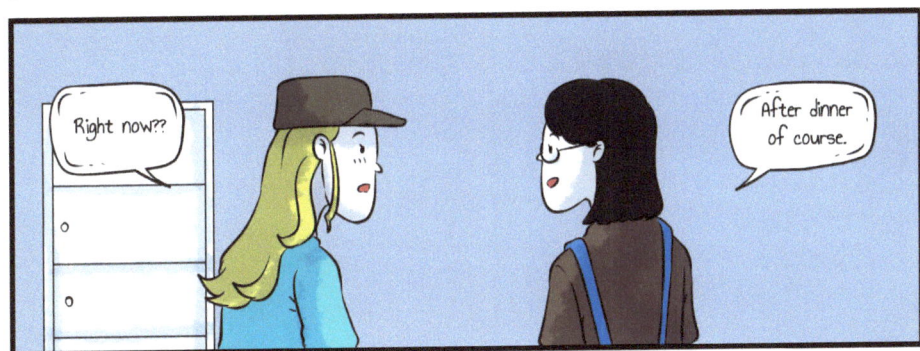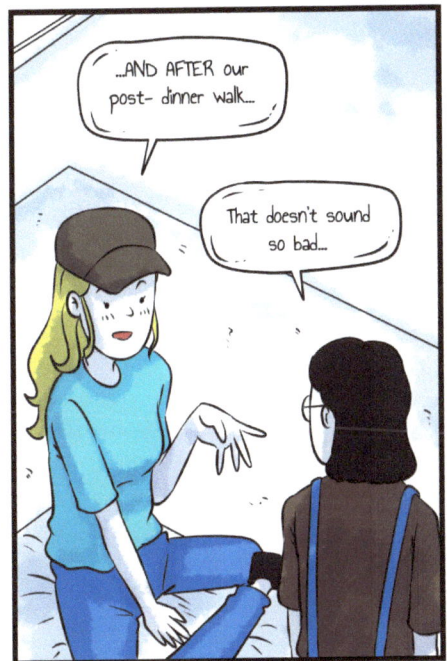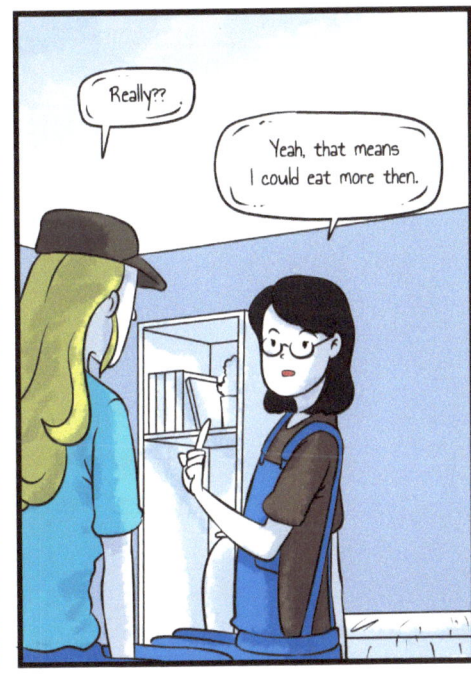

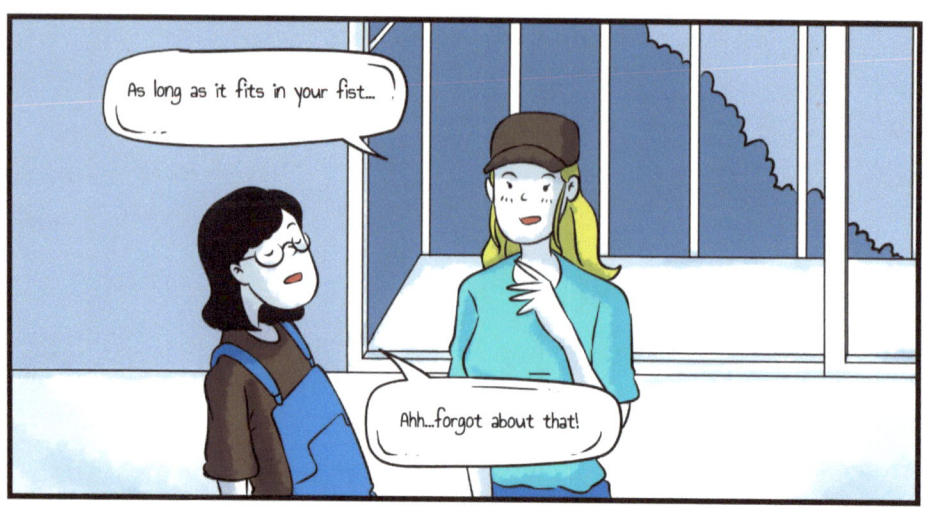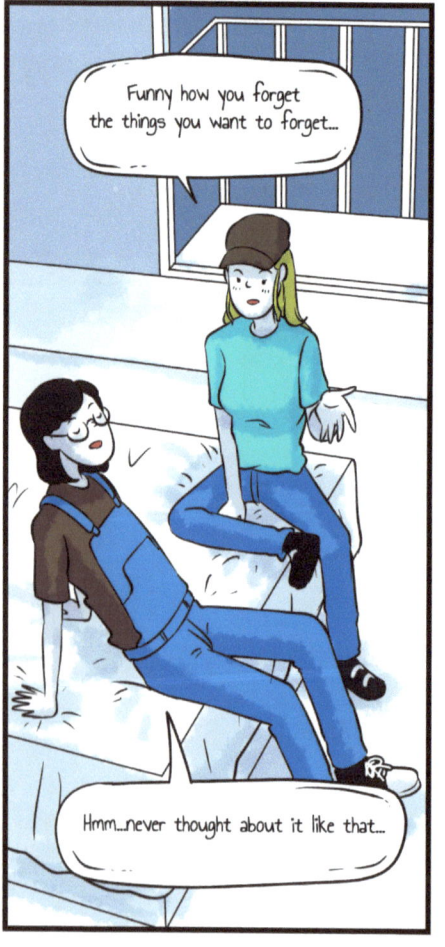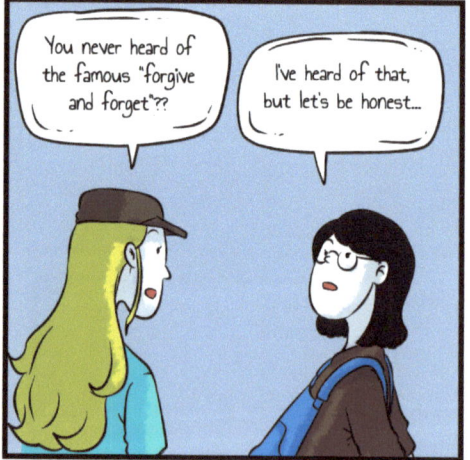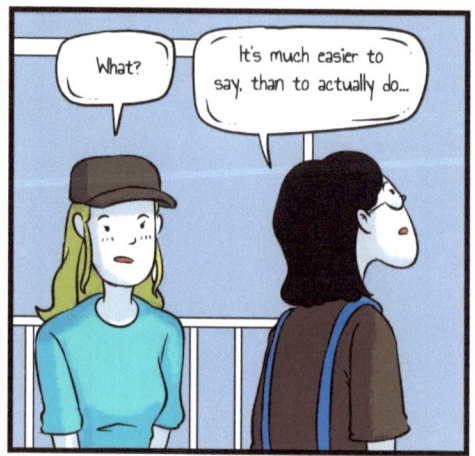

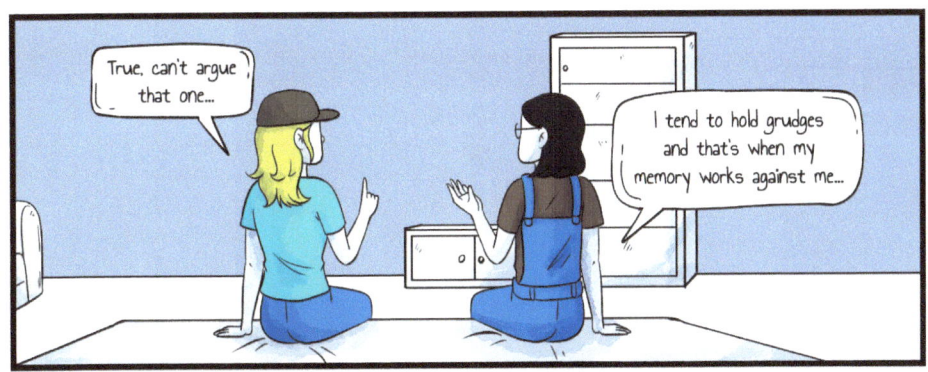
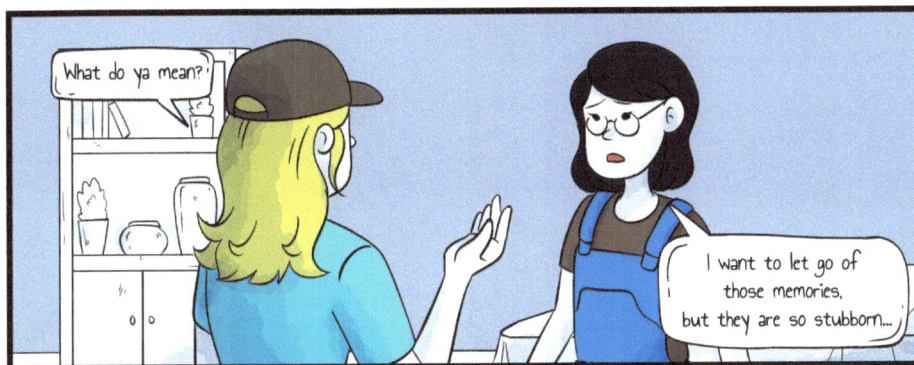
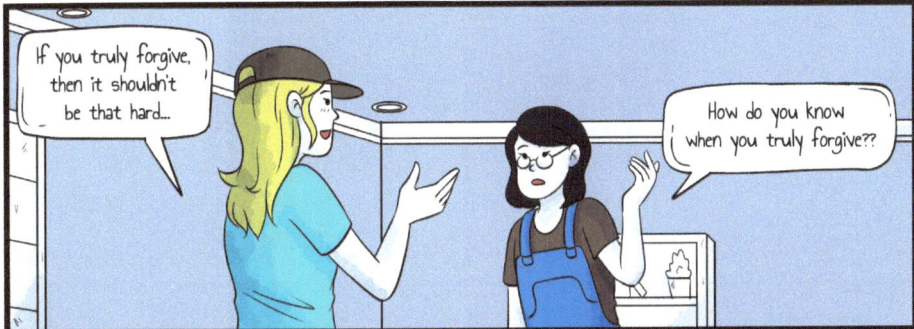
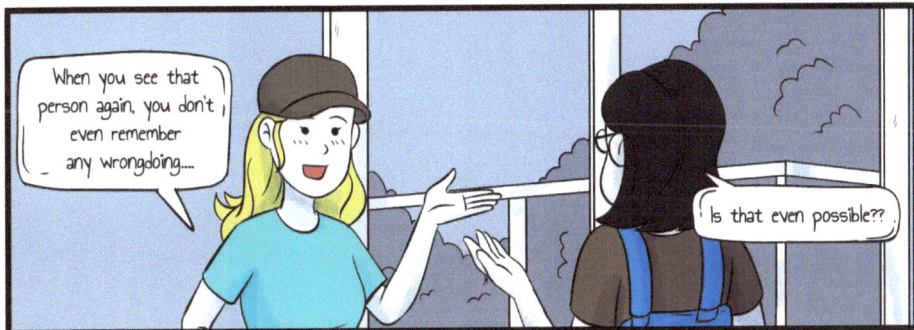

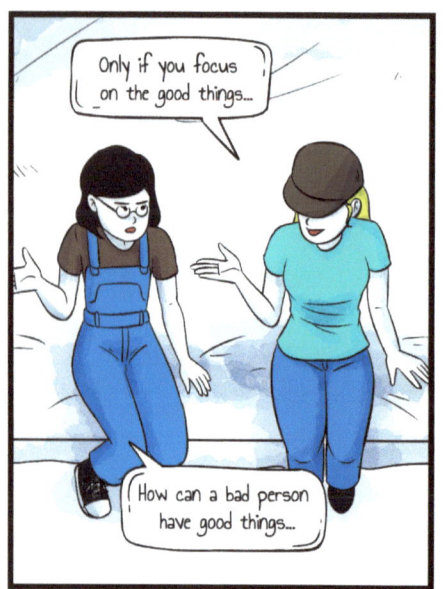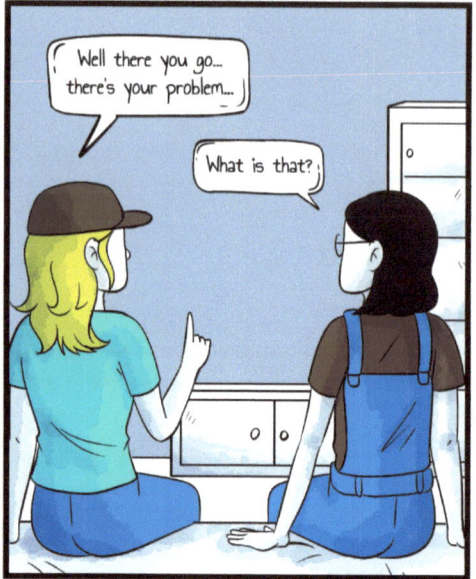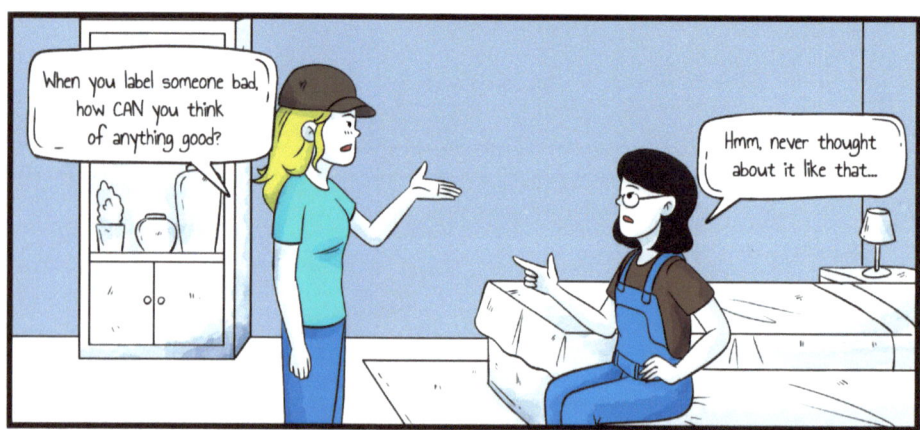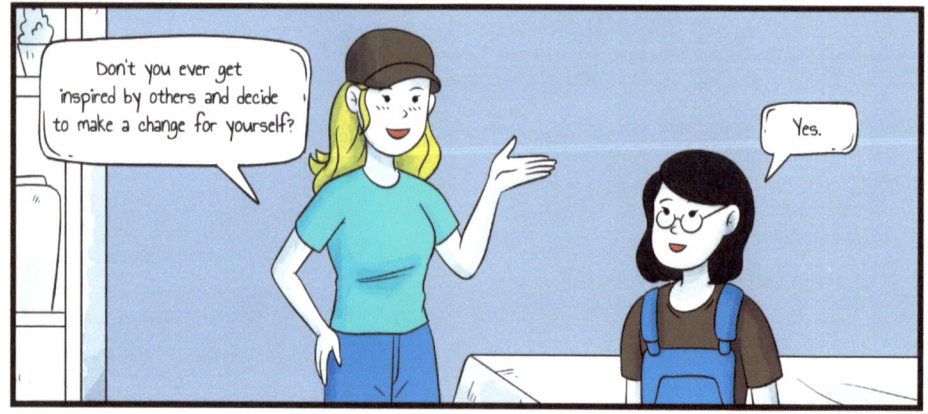

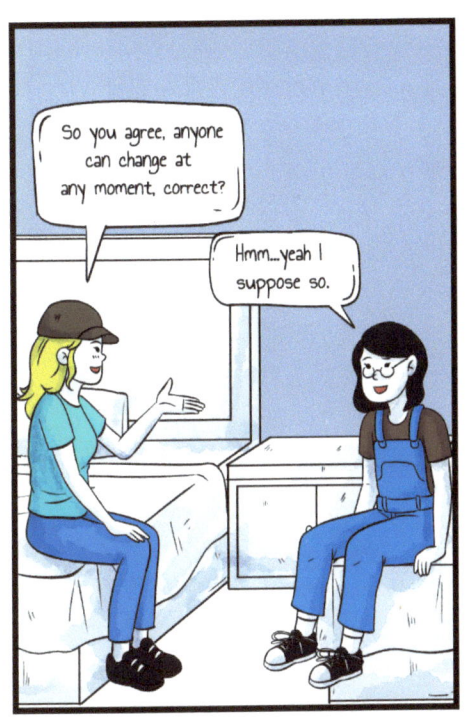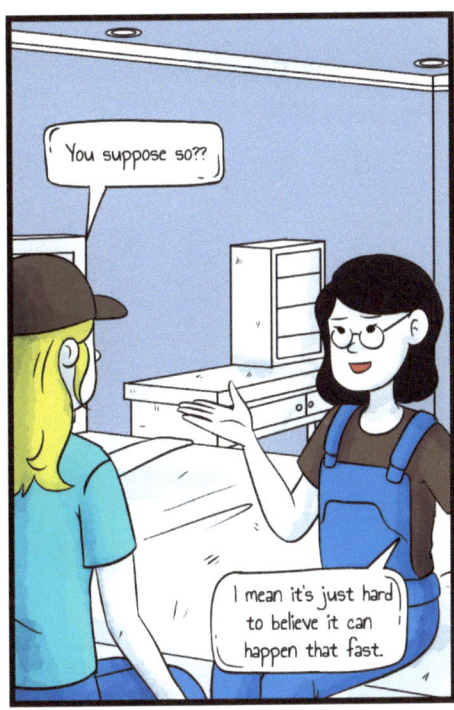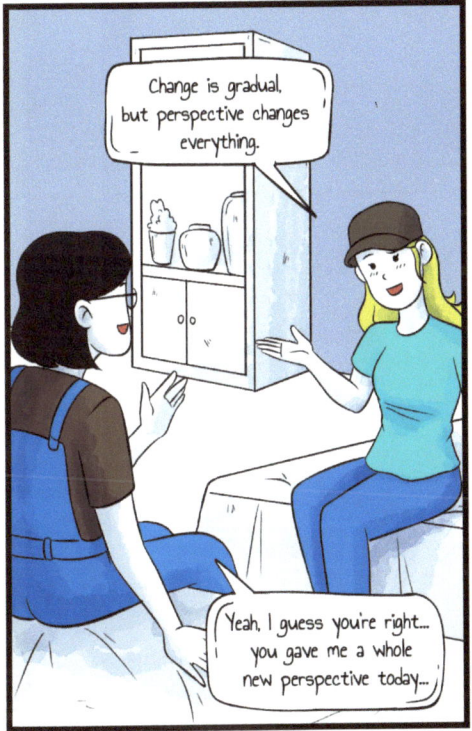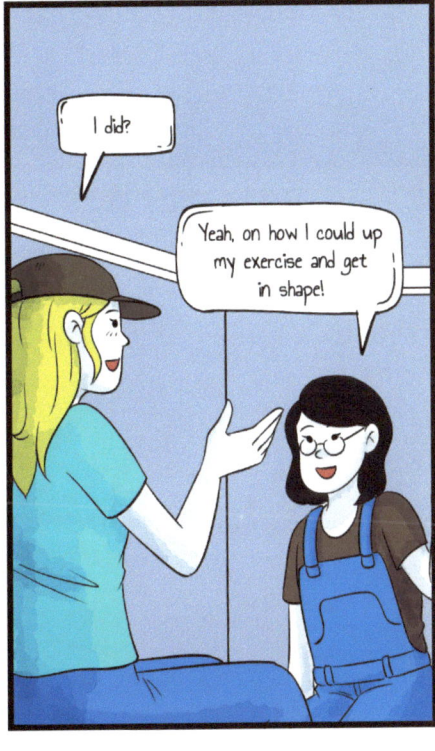

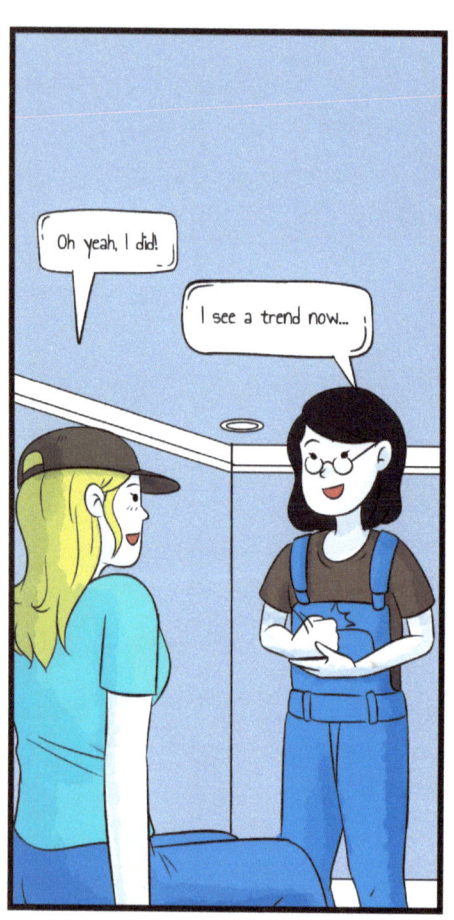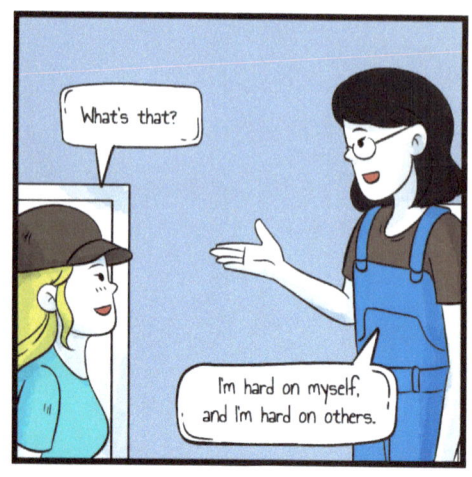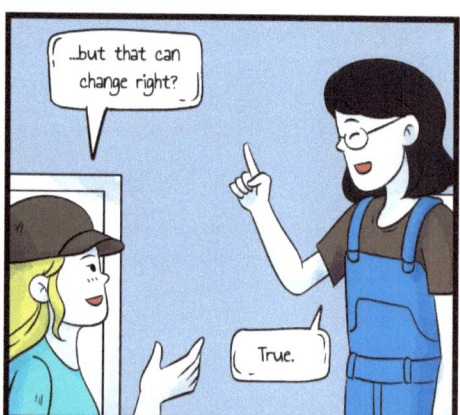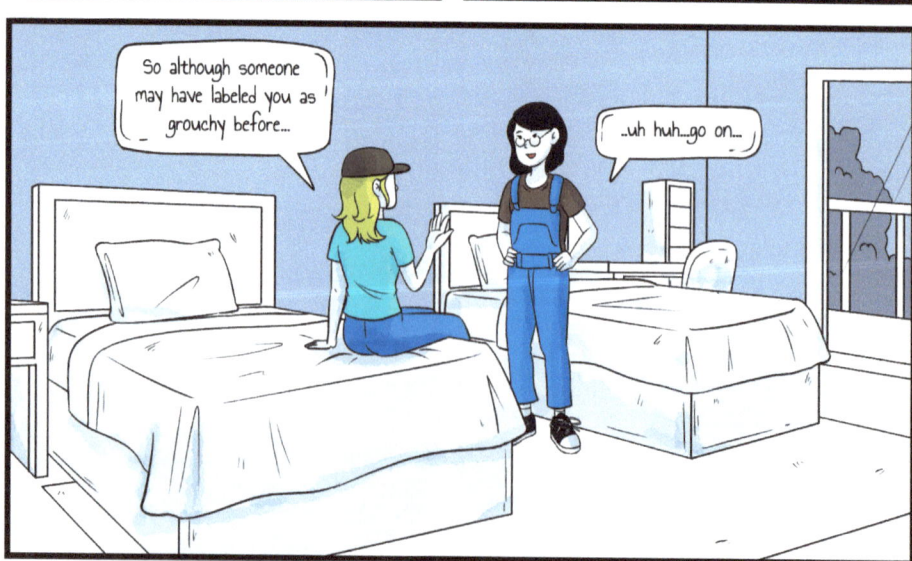

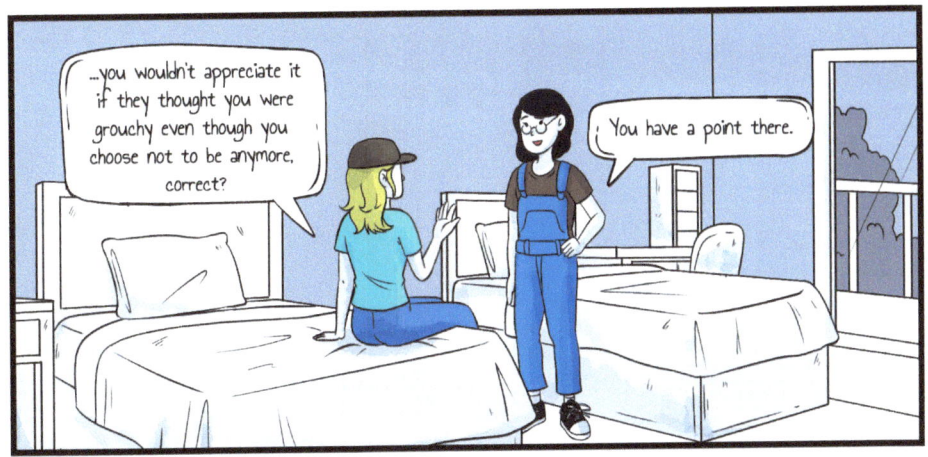

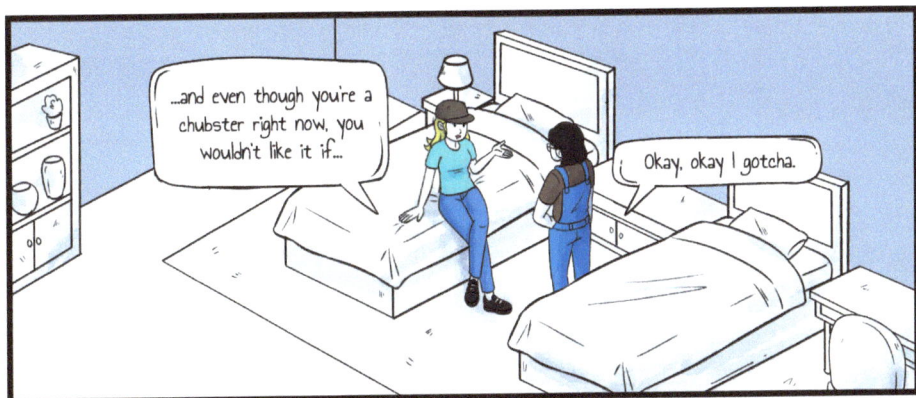

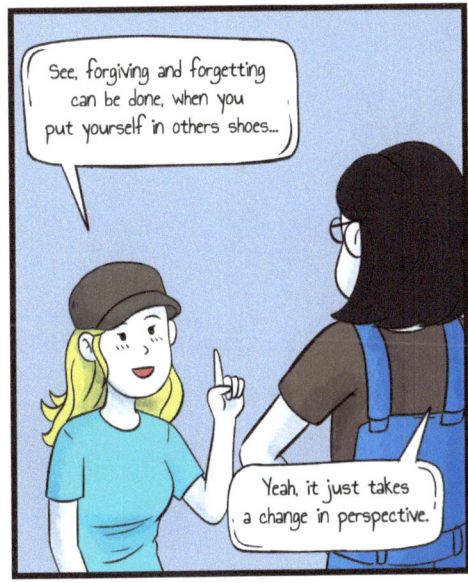

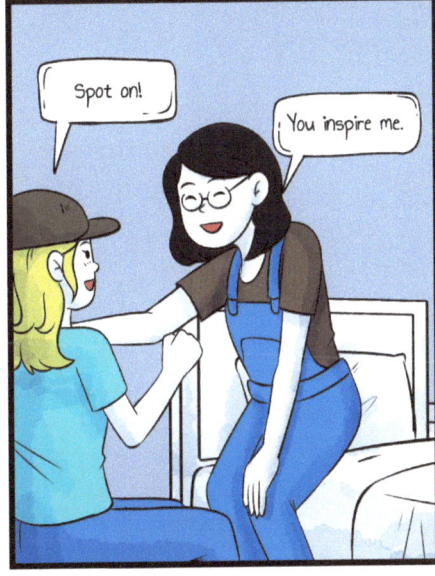

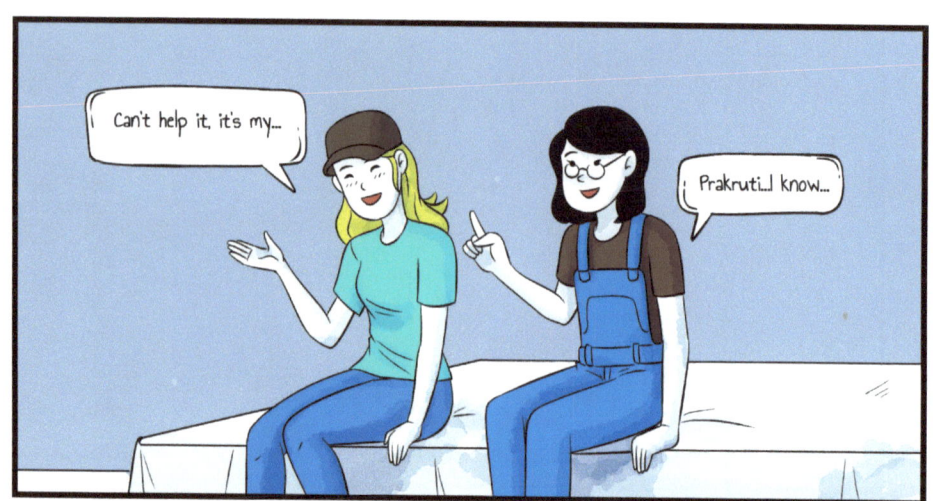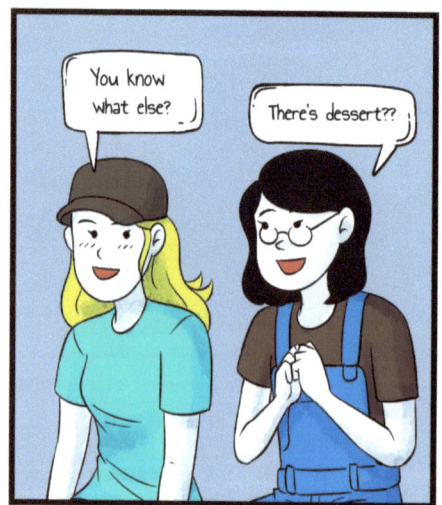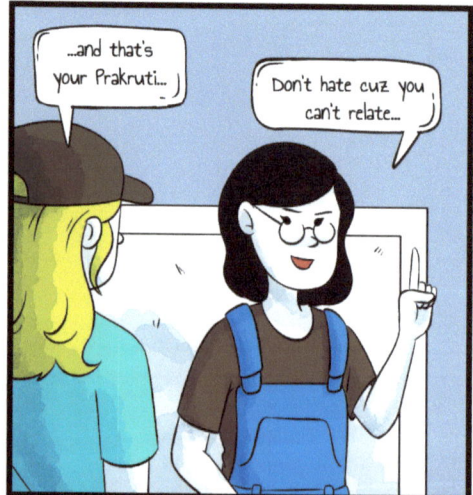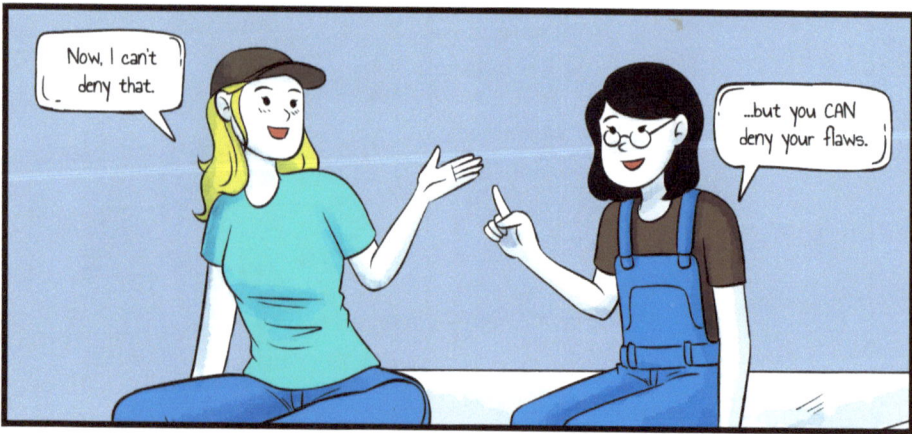

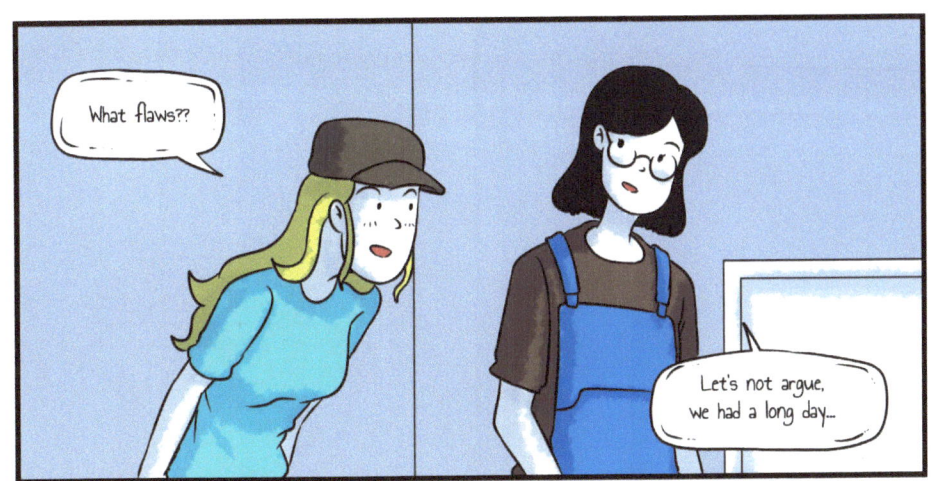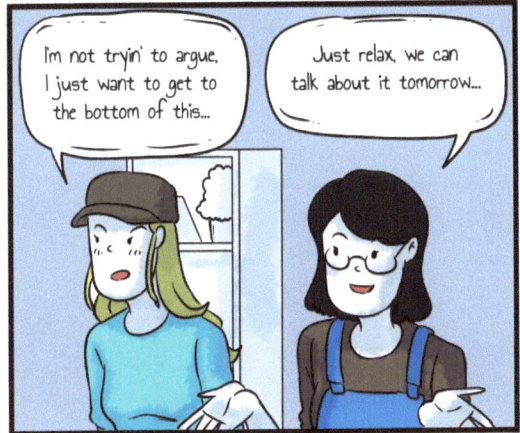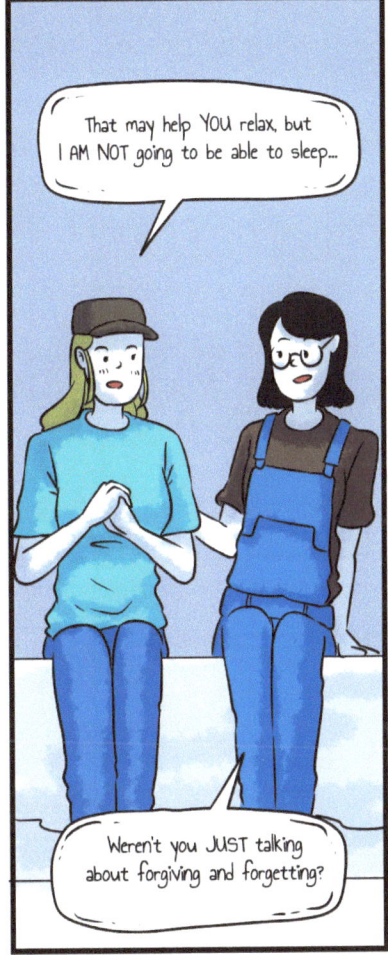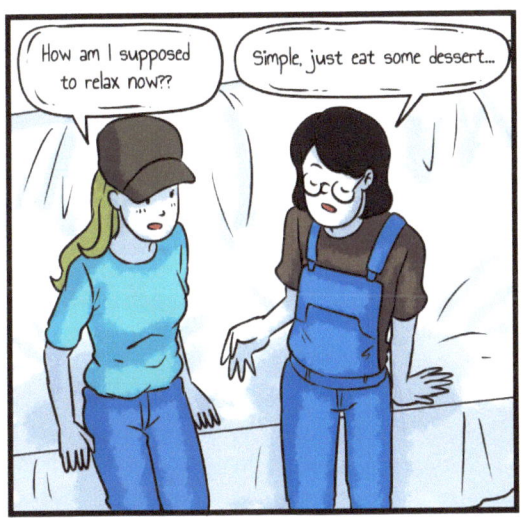

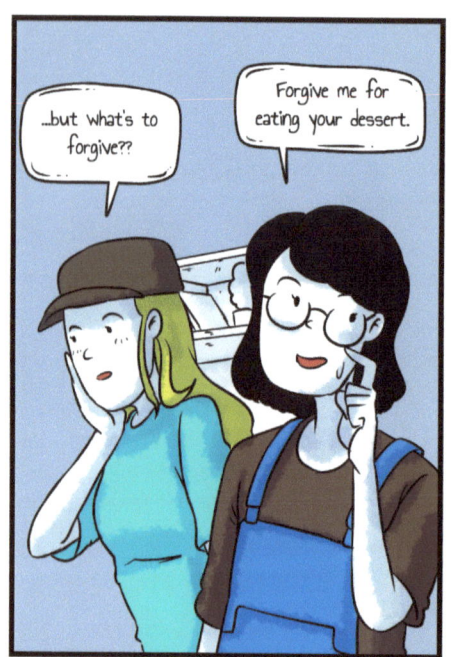
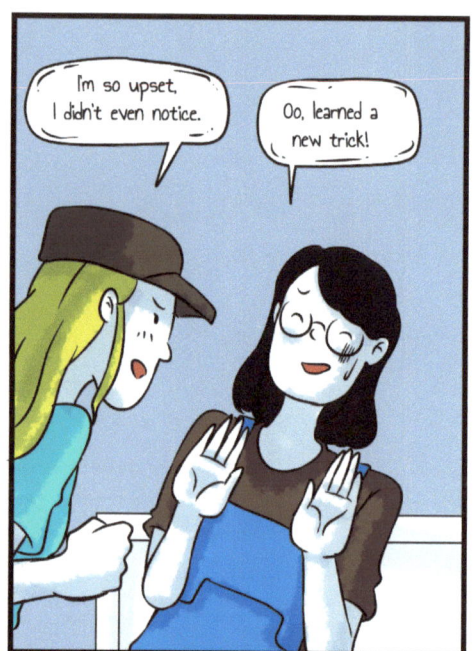
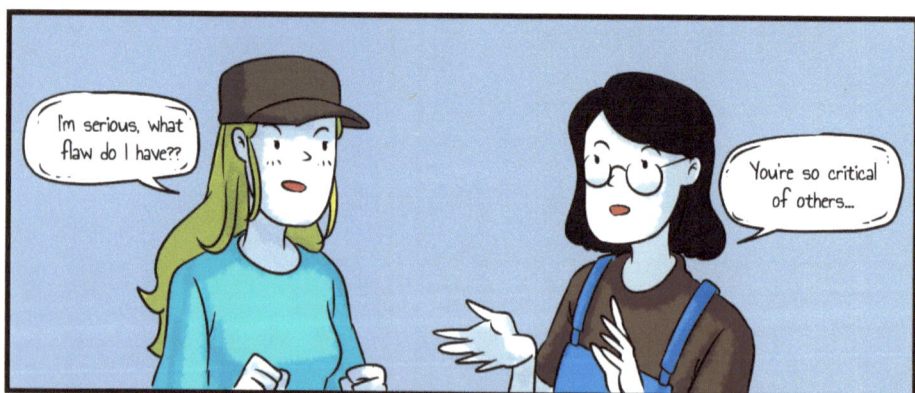
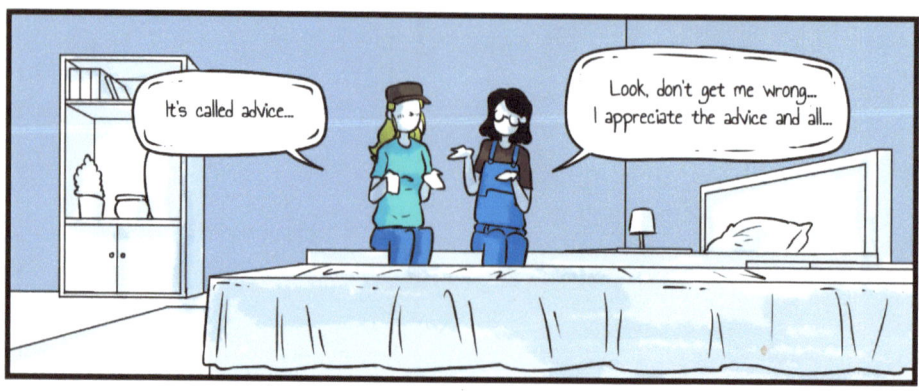

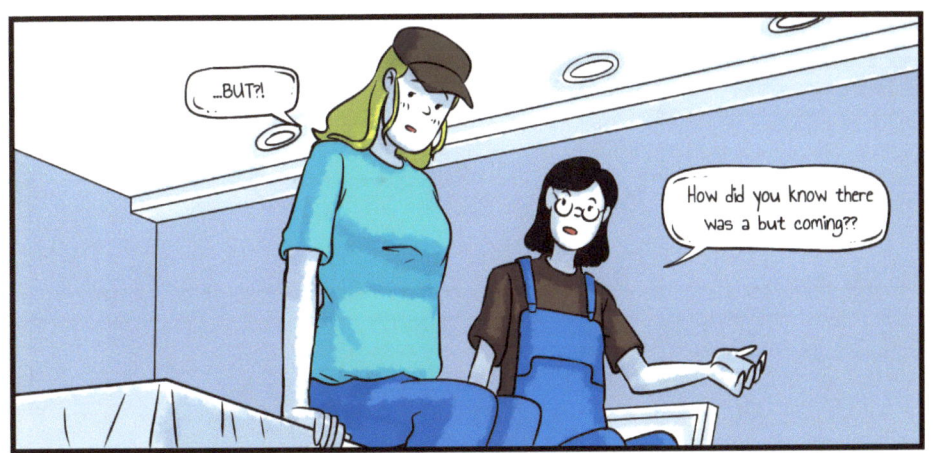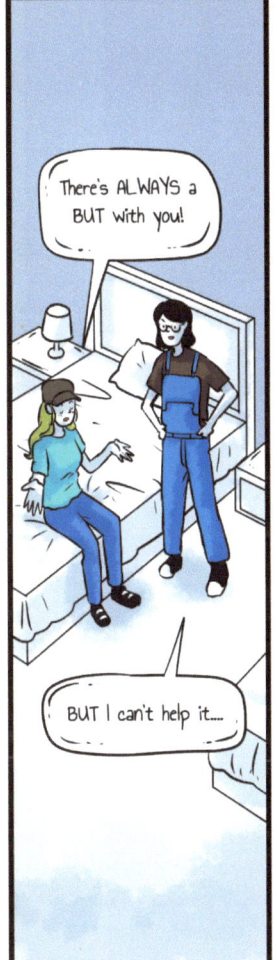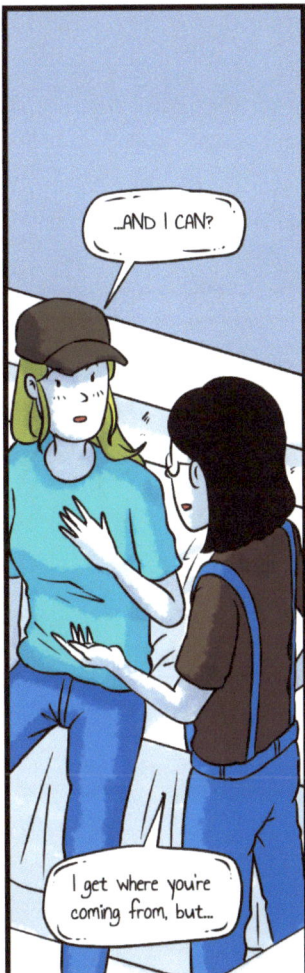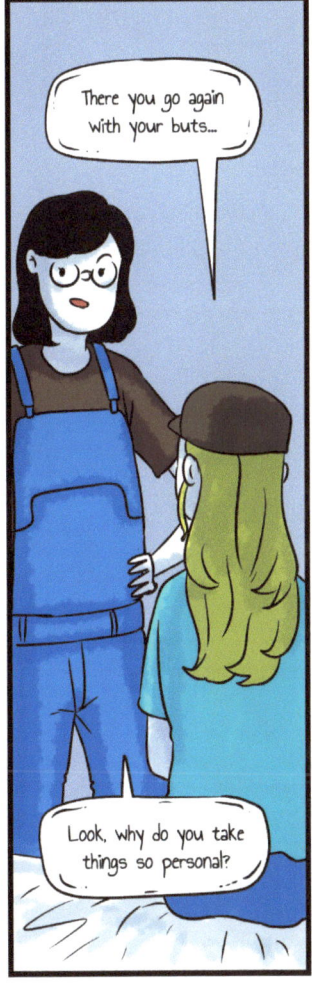

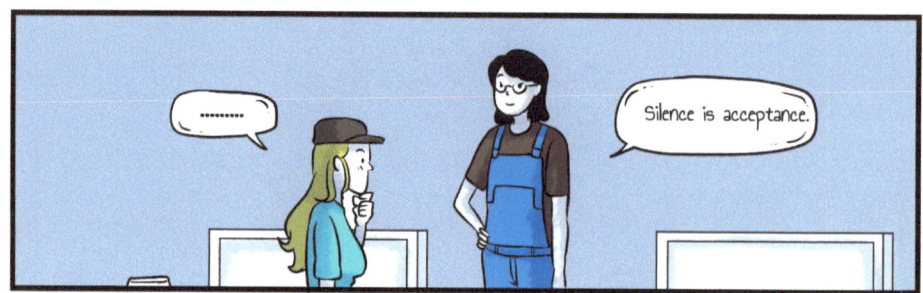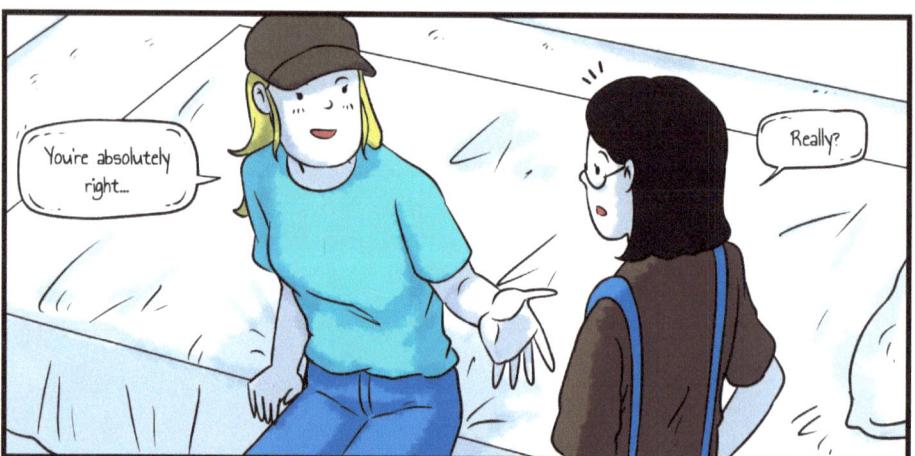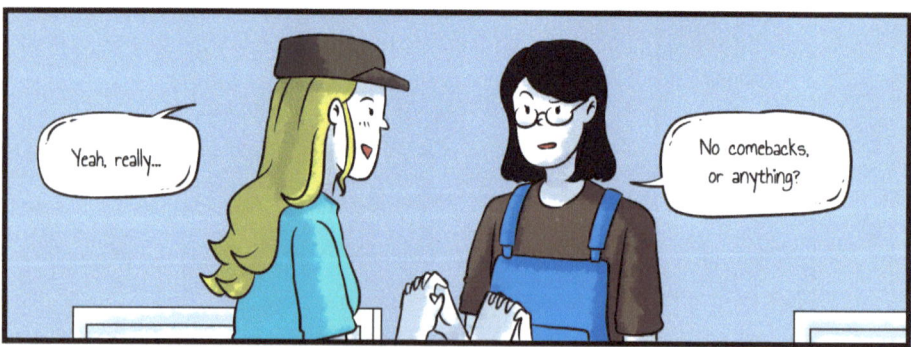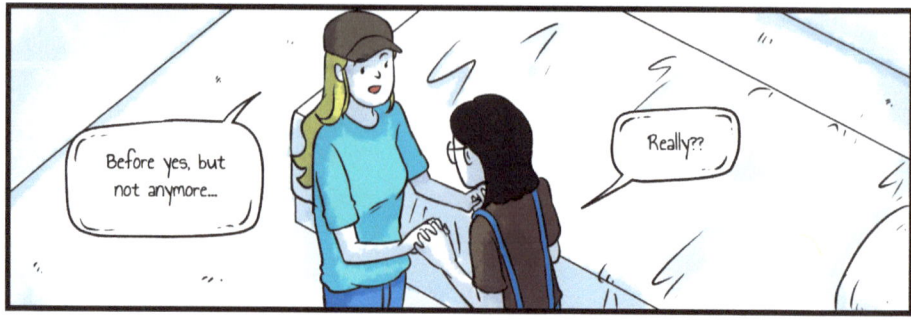

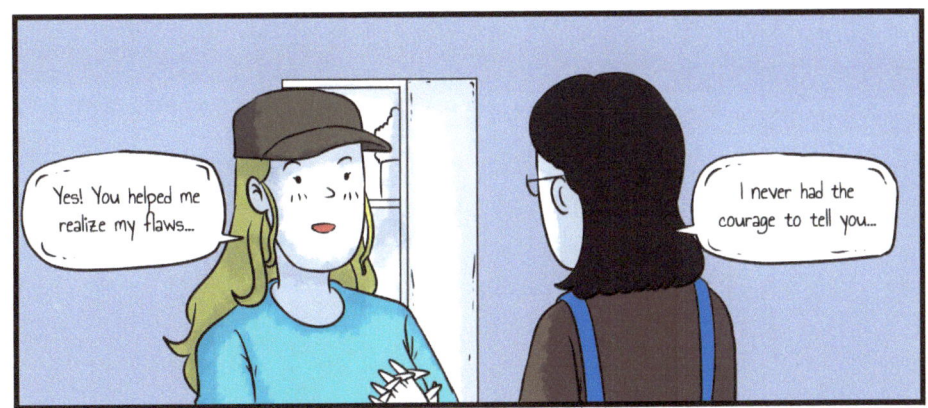

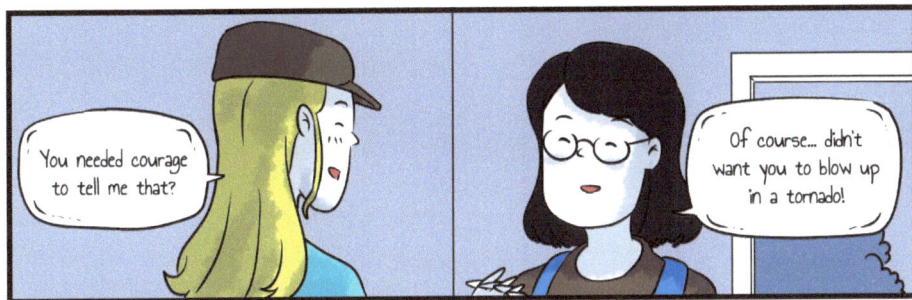

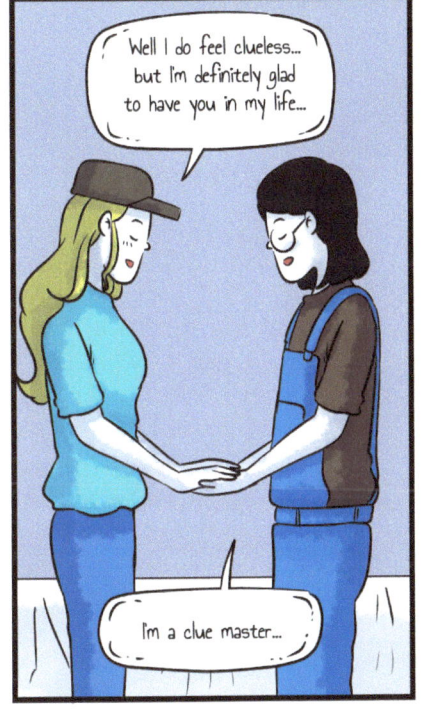

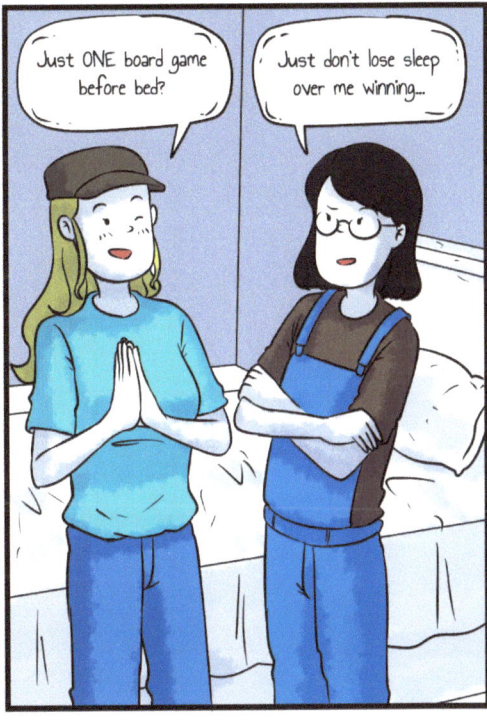

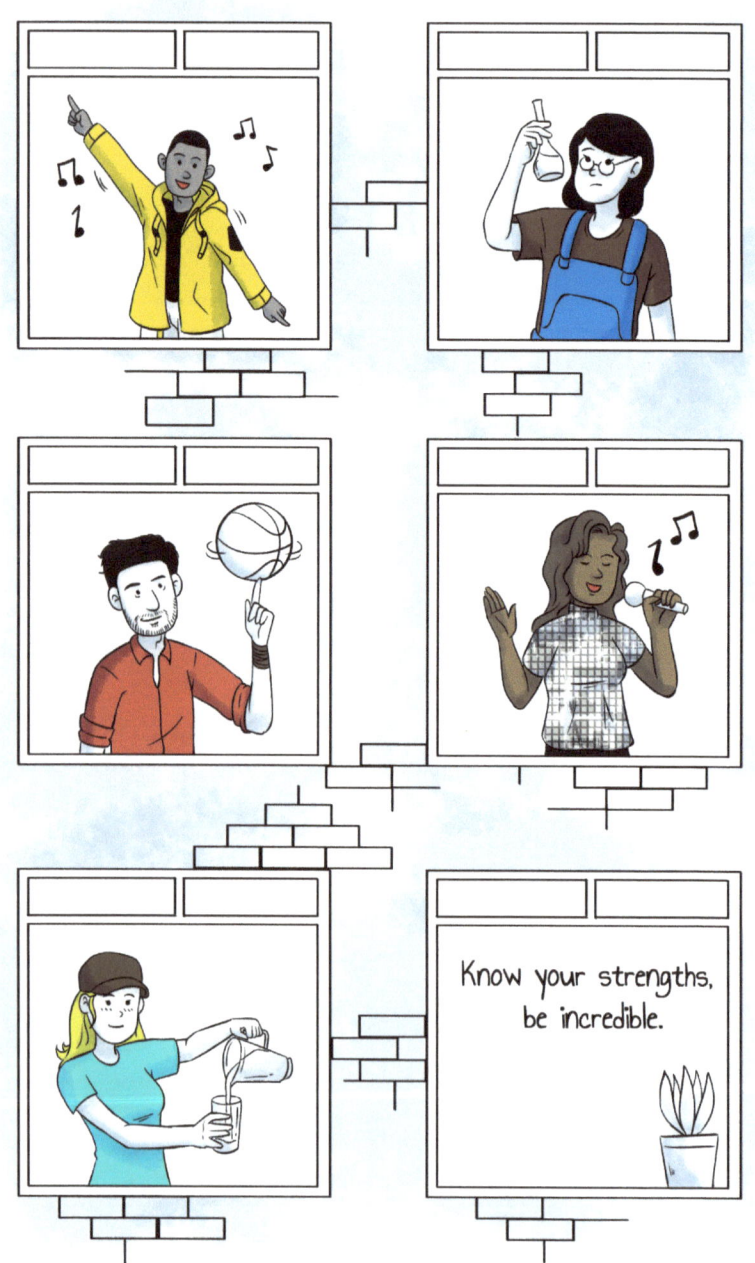

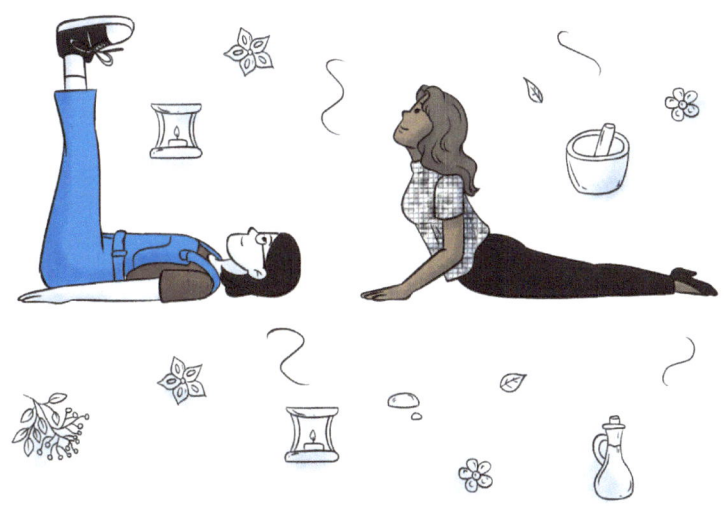

Rule #1 Good intentions are magical
Rule #2 Control your emotions to control your life
Rule #3 Perspective is everything

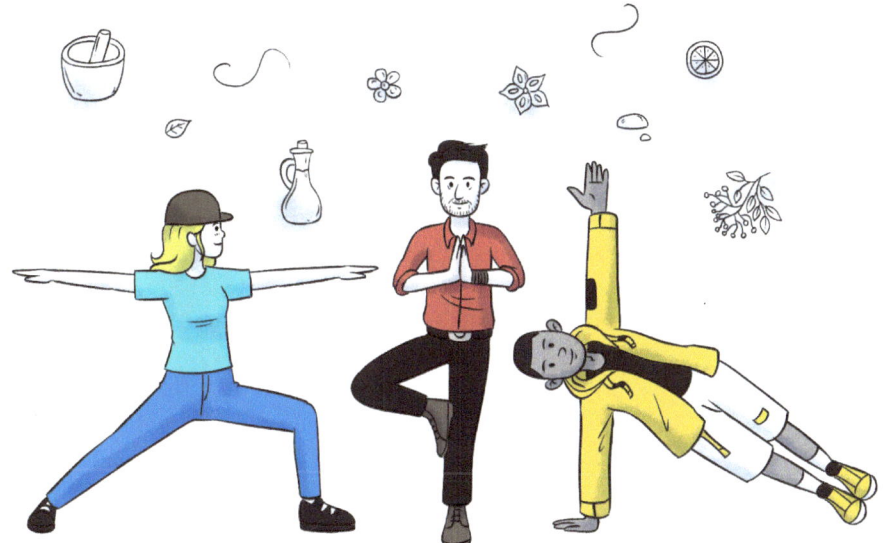

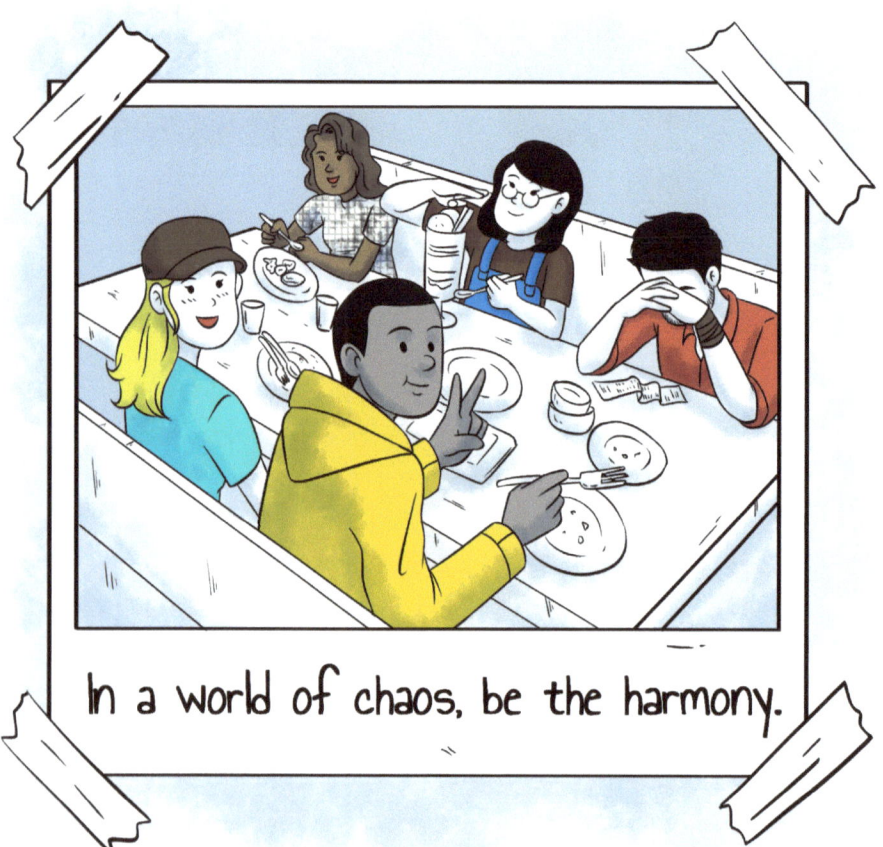

www.ingramcontent.com/pod-product-compliance
Lightning Source LLC
Chambersburg PA
CBHW040317220526
45473CB00009B/2463